EDITORS' FOREWORD

The scope of this series has increased since it was first established, and it now serves a wide range of medical, nursing and ancillary professions, in line with the present trend towards the belief that all who care for patients in a clinical context have an increasing amount in common.

The texts are carefully prepared and organised so that they may be readily kept up to date as the rapid developments of medical science demand. The series already includes many popular books on various aspects of medical and nursing care, and reflects the increased emphasis on community care.

The increasing specialisation in the medical profession is fully appreciated and the books are often written by physicians or surgeons in conjunction with specialist nurses. For this reason, they will not only cover the syllabus of training of the General Nursing Council, but will be designed to meet the needs of those undertaking trainings controlled by the Joint Board of Clinical Studies.

PATHOLOGY

C. P. MAYERS
M.B., Ch.B., M.R.C.Path

HODDER AND STOUGHTON
LONDON   SYDNEY   AUCKLAND   TORONTO

ISBN 0 340 22397 9

First Printed 1972
Reprinted 1975
Second edition 1977
Reprinted 1979, 1982

Printed and bound in Great Britain
for Hodder and Stoughton Educational,
a division of Hodder and Stoughton Ltd,
Mill Road, Dunton Green, Sevenoaks, Kent
by Biddles Ltd, Guildford, Surrey

AUTHOR'S PREFACE

Pathology is about diseases and disease processes. This book has been written to give nurses and nursing students a short account of the common disease processes and their causes and effects. It is hoped that this will help them to understand and derive satisfaction from their work. It may also assist them to understand the distress of patients who have physical ailments.

The requirements of nurses are different from those of doctors, and so there is little here about the diagnosis or treatment of diseases, or about their microscopic appearances. I have, however, mentioned some recent advances, especially in the fields of cancer research and atherosclerosis.

General disease processes such as inflammation and cancer are described in the first half of the book, and the diseases affecting each of the various bodily systems are described in the second half. The choice of topics is based partly on the examination requirements of the Nursing Councils in Great Britain, Canada and Australia and partly on my experience in hospital wards, in general practice, as a lecturer in pathology and as a director of hospital laboratories. All the errors, oversimplifications and omissions are mine.

There is nothing in this book about Obstetrics and Gynaecology, Psychology and Psychiatry or about Neurology as these topics are very ably covered in other books in this series. There are, however, brief descriptions of some of the commoner tropical diseases.

This book is based on lecture courses given in the Nursing Studies Department of Edinburgh University. I am grateful to Professor G. L. Montgomery, Head of the Department of Pathology, and to the late Miss E. Stephenson and Professor Margaret Scott Wright, Directors, and Miss K. J. W. Wilson, Acting Director of the Nursing Studies Department for asking me to organise the lecture courses, and I am grateful to several years of Nurse-Teacher students for their questions and comments. I am also grateful to my colleagues in the Pathology Department for their helpful comments and criticisms; to Mrs Rigg and the Secretaries of the Pathology Department and Miss M. Todd for their careful typing; to Professor A. J. H. Rains and Miss Valerie Hunt, General Editors of this series, and to Mr B. Steven of Hodder and Stoughton Educational for their interest and guidance.

NOTE TO SECOND EDITION

Our knowledge of disease processes has advanced since the first edition in 1972. The new SI (Système Internationale) units of measurement have been introduced, and other new items in this edition include T and B lymphocytes, new information about chemical carcinogens, HBsAg, thyroid stimulators and histocompatibility antigens in ankylosing spondylitis.

CONTENTS

1 *DISTURBANCES OF THE INTERNAL ENVIRONMENT*

WATER BALANCE
Dehydration

ELECTROLYTES
Sodium
Potassium

ACID-BASE DISTURBANCE

RESPONSES TO STRESS

The cells of the body are constantly immersed in fluid, the extracellular fluid. The cells are entirely dependent upon it for their supplies and maintenance. The extracellular fluid constitutes the internal environment of the body and the cells are affected by any change in its volume or composition.

In this chapter we shall consider some of the ways in which the internal environment may be disturbed. The changes we shall consider are those of water volume, of salt concentration and of acidity. For greater simplicity, the changes are described one at a time, as though water, salts and acidity were independent of each other, but in reality they are intimately interconnected. Changes affecting other important qualities of the internal environment, such as temperature and oxygen concentration, will be dealt with in later chapters.

WATER BALANCE

Water is the principal constituent of the body. It accounts for two-thirds of the weight of the body. An average man weighs 70 kg and contains about 45 litres of water, that is about 75 pints.

In temperate climates, we drink about 1·5 litres of water a day. There is about another litre of water in the food we eat, and a further 0·5 litre of water is produced by the oxidation of food. So on average, we have a daily intake of about 3 litres of water. This intake, in most people, is controlled by the sensation of thirst, which is a remarkably accurate guide to our water requirements. Deficient intake is therefore seldom seen, but it does occur in infants, unconscious patients or patients who are too ill or otherwise incapable of demanding water.

There is a tremendous turnover of water each day in the gastrointestinal tract. It is estimated that, in an adult, about 10 litres of fluid are passed into the gut each day in the form of saliva, gastric, pancreatic and other secretions. Normally nearly

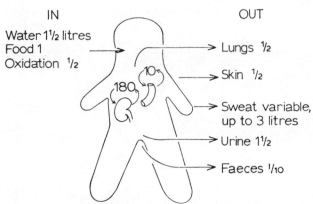

IN

Water 1½ litres
Food 1
Oxidation ½

OUT

Lungs ½
Skin ½
Sweat variable,
up to 3 litres
Urine 1½
Faeces ¹/₁₀

FIG. 1-1 Water balance man. Normal turnover rates of water in litres per day

all of this fluid is reabsorbed by the colon, and only about 0·1 litre is lost in the faeces. In any condition in which this reabsorption does not take place, dehydration may occur. Cholera is the most dramatic of these conditions, and 5 or more litres may be lost in a day. Other conditions in which large volumes of water may be lost include severe vomiting, diarrhoea and dysentery.

The two kidneys between them have an even greater turnover of water each day, amounting to 180 litres. This vast amount of fluid passes out of the blood through the membranes of the kidney glomeruli and is then reabsorbed from the kidney tubules. This reabsorption is partially controlled by the antidiuretic hormone formed in the posterior part of the pituitary gland. Thus, either kidney disease, or less commonly posterior pituitary disease, may result in large urine volumes, and this requires a large water intake to make up for it.

Sweating may account for up to 3 litres or more of water output a day. This loss, if uncorrected, produces dehydration and this is an important factor in producing heat exhaustion. The amount lost by sweating varies very much depending on the needs of temperature control.

Normally only about 0·5 litre per day is lost by unseen evaporation through the skin as the skin forms an effective barrier to water loss. The loss occurs whatever the air temperature. If the skin is damaged, however, the barrier is impaired, and then the fluid loss may be considerable. Thus in superficial burns, and even with quite a mild sunburn, the skin loss may be increased.

Another 0·5 litre per day is lost through the lungs. This figure must be allowed for in any calculations of fluid balance, but it is not noticeably altered in lung disease.

Dehydration

We have seen that dehydration may result from a deficient intake of water, or from an excessive output, from the intestines, the kidneys or the skin. Sometimes dehydration is due to a combination of deficient intake and excessive output.

Severe dehydration is seen in cholera. The patients have shrunken tissues, with wrinkled washerwomen's fingers, sunken eyeballs, thirst, dry tongues, low urine outputs, and weakness or coma due to low blood pressure.

Less severe forms of dehydration are commoner. For instance, patients with ileostomies tend to have very watery faeces, and they may be mildly but chronically short of water. And most of us have had personal experience of diarrhoea or severe sunburn, and also of the aftermath of fatigue and weakness which is largely due to the dehydration produced by these conditions.

Excessive water intake is seldom seen, as most people are capable of getting rid of any excess via the kidneys. Water intoxication can however occur, due to over-zealous transfusion. It occurs, for instance, in patients with poor kidney function if they are given excessive glucose transfusions. It also occurs occasionally in small infants given too much to drink, as infants have a less efficient control mechanism than adults.

In general though, dehydration is much commoner than excess of water. Nearly everyone can dispose of an excess, but not everyone can ensure an intake adequate for their needs.

ELECTROLYTES

The body fluids contain various salts dissolved in water. When dissolved, the salt molecules tend to separate into individual particles, each carrying a small electrical charge, some positive and some negative. Substances which have such electrical charges in solution are called electrolytes. Their concentrations are measured in mille-moles per litre (mmol/l). The electrolytes we shall mention are sodium (Na^+) and potassium (K^+).

SODIUM

Sodium in the body is found in the blood and in the extracellular fluid, and it can readily be measured. The normal level is 135-150 mmol/l. There is very little sodium within the body cells. The amount of sodium in the body is largely controlled by a hormone called aldosterone, made in the cortex of the adrenal gland. The less sodium we get in our food, the more aldosterone is secreted, and the more sodium is reabsorbed by the kidney tubules from the glomerular filtrate.

Most of the body secretions contain a fair amount of sodium. Thus loss of secretions, such as sweat, or of intestinal fluid in diarrhoea, depletes the body of both sodium and water. If this loss is great, the volume of the extracellular fluid and of the blood is decreased, and the blood pressure falls. The patient is in shock, with weakness and muscle cramps. It may be noted that in such cases, when water and sodium are both lost together, the concentration of the sodium in the blood is often normal.

If, however, the lost water is replaced by drinking, then the sodium loss shows in the reduced blood sodium level. The classic demonstration of this occurs in miners who sweat a lot, losing water and sodium. If they replace their losses by drinking only beer or water, they suffer muscle cramps due to sodium deficiency. To remedy this, they put salt in their beer, and this works very well.

Sodium deficiencies can also occur in some cases of kidney disease such as sodium-losing nephritis, and also in adrenal insufficiency (Addison's disease) due to aldosterone deficiency.

High sodium levels are seldom due to excess sodium intake as most people can dispose of any excess simply by not reabsorbing sodium from the kidney tubules. Sodium excess is therefore not caused by excess intake, but it can be caused by excessive production of aldosterone, which causes excessive sodium retention. This occurs in some tumours of the adrenal cortex, and is known as aldosteronism. The excess sodium tends to encourage more water to stay in the body. The consequent increased volume of extracellular fluid shows as oedema, and the increased blood volume shows as an increase in blood pressure. Indeed, aldosteronism is one of the causes of high blood pressure, particularly in young patients. A similar but more moderate rise in the level of aldosterone occurs in patients with failing hearts, and in pregnancy, and they may show sodium retention, oedema and sometimes raised blood pressure.

POTASSIUM

Potassium is found mainly in the cells. It is difficult to measure intracellular potassium properly, so usually we measure the small amount of potassium outside the

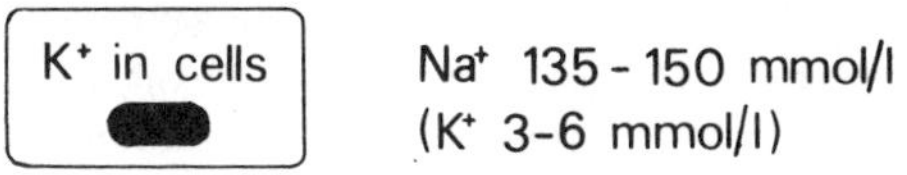

| K⁺ in cells | Na⁺ 135 - 150 mmol/l |
| | (K⁺ 3-6 mmol/l) |

FIG. 1-2 A cell and the normal levels of the electrolytes outside the cell

cells, in the blood. This gives an approximate guide to the state of affairs inside the cells. If the potassium comes out of the cells, the level of the potassium in the blood rises, and we can measure it. This happens in cases of biochemical injury to the cells, such as in aspirin poisoning or diabetic ketosis, and it may happen in other kinds of cell injury. (Potassium also comes out of red blood cells if they are damaged, which is one reason why laboratories do not like haemolysed blood samples for testing.)

Potassium deficiency is not common, as we all have large stores of potassium in all the cells of our bodies, and also we take in potassium in the cells we eat, such as in meat or vegetables. But potassium deficiency does sometimes occur, especially if there is a persistent loss of mucus from the body. Mucus is rich in potassium, and potassium deficiency may occur in patients who vomit persistently, or lose mucus by gastric suction. Not only do they lose mucus but they have little potassium intake. If this continues, they suffer potassium deficiency and they show confusion, weakness, ileus and changes in their electrocardiographic patterns.

ACID-BASE DISTURBANCE

The cells of the body continuously produce acids of various kinds that must be disposed of via the lungs or kidneys.

These acids are:
- (a) *Carbon dioxide*—a gas which can dissolve in water to form carbonic acid, and which can be turned back into gas and be 'blown off' in the lungs.
- (b) *Organic acids*—such as lactic acid, which can eventually be turned into carbon dioxide, and disposed of by the lungs.
- (c) *Inorganic acids*—such as sulphuric acid, which can only be excreted by the kidneys.

The first stage in dealing with these acids is to transport them to the lungs or kidneys. To do this, there are various substances in the blood which act as buffers— that is they 'soak up' the acidity so that the acids can be safely transported. These buffer systems are very effective, and they can 'soak up' a large amount of acid without there being any change in the acidity. One effect of this is that a measure of the acidity of the blood is a very poor guide to the quantity of acid present. It is much more useful to measure how much carbon dioxide is present in the blood (normal level 36-44 mm of mercury) and also whether the buffers have been changed by 'soaking up' acid (measured as bicarbonate, normal level 22-28 mmol/l, as CO_2 combining power).

The second stage in dealing with the acids is their removal, by the lungs in the case of carbon dioxide, or by the kidneys in the case of inorganic acids. It is this second stage that may be upset by diseases of the lungs or kidneys.

Lung disease, for instance, causes an accumulation of carbon dioxide in the blood.

Hypoventilation or the depressing action of morphine on the respiratory control centre have the same effect. The rise of the carbon dioxide in the blood can be measured. In an attempt to make up for the failure of the lungs, the kidneys may excrete more inorganic acid than usual, and they make more bicarbonate, and this shows in the bicarbonate measurements. The patient in this situation would probably show other changes as well, such as laboured breathing and a low blood oxygen level. This state of affairs is referred to as respiratory acidosis, although, as already mentioned, due to the action of the buffers the actual acidity of the blood hardly changes, even though excess acid is present. The buffer systems work very well, but they may become overloaded, if for instance the lung disease becomes more severe. Then the acidity really does change and the patient may die.

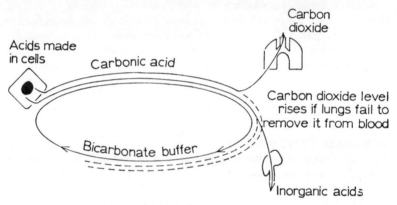

Fig. 1-3   Acid-base balance, showing how changes may occur in diseases of the lungs or kidneys

The opposite picture, known as respiratory alkalosis, can occur if a patient breathes too much, and 'blows off' more than the normal quantity of carbon dioxide. This can occur due to anxiety or hysteria, or occasionally due to excessive use of artificial respiration apparatus.

In kidney disease, the kidneys fail to excrete inorganic acids, and they do not make bicarbonate. The lungs may attempt to compensate; this is seen as air-hunger and the blood carbon dioxide level is low. This condition is known as renal acidosis. Measurements in this condition show low bicarbonate levels and low carbon dioxide levels. These patients tend also to have high blood potassium levels.

Metabolic alkalosis occurs principally in ulcer patients. They may repeatedly lose gastric acid, by vomiting or via a stomach tube, or they may continuously suck alkali tablets. These patients may have shallow breathing which results in retention of carbonic acid, a respiratory compensation for the metabolic alkalosis. These patients often also have low potassium levels, due to the potassium lost in the gastric mucus.

Here are examples of the chemical measurements that might be made in two common kinds of disease:

(a) *Lung disease* such as emphysema may cause a retention of carbon dioxide in the body, a respiratory acidosis in which the blood carbon dioxide level would be above 44 mm Hg, and the buffers would be altered by taking up more acid than usual so the carbon dioxide combining power would be reduced to below 22 mmol/l.

(b) In *kidney disease*, the kidneys may fail to excrete inorganic acids and this causes renal acidosis. In this case the buffers would be altered by taking up more acid than usual and this would be reflected by a low carbon dioxide combining power (below 22 mmol/l). Provided the lungs were healthy, the blood carbon dioxide level would be normal (36-44 mm Hg), or even reduced by respiratory compensation.

RESPONSES TO STRESS

Any kind of stress produces a constant pattern of chemical changes in the internal environment. These include retention of sodium and of water in the body due to increased aldosterone production, and loss of potassium from the cells into the extracellular fluid and blood. There is also a breakdown of cell protein and loss of some of the protein nitrogen in the urine. These changes occur after surgical operations, in severe infections and in fact in almost any kind of stress or injury. For instance, a patient with burns, in addition to the marked loss of fluid from the damaged skin area already mentioned, will show the chemical changes described above, in response to stress. These changes cannot be prevented by treatment, and they are considered to be the normal responses of the body to abnormal attacks upon it.

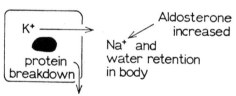

FIG. 1-4 Stress. The chemical changes that occur as a reaction to any kind of stress

2 INFLAMMATION AND REPAIR

REACTION TO INJURY

CHANGES IN BLOOD FLOW
Increase of Capillary Permeability
The Fluid Exudate
The Inflammatory Cells
Changes in Tissue Cells

Mechanisms of Inflammation

GENERALISED BODY CHANGES

EVENTS FOLLOWING INFLAMMATION
Repair

Chronic Inflammation

REACTION TO INJURY

If I step on a splinter, my foot may become inflamed. My foot may also become inflamed if I drop a rock on it, or leave it out in the sun too long, or drop concentrated acid on it, or infect it with bacteria or damage it in any other way. Whatever the injury, inflammation may occur. It would be pointless to list all the different possible causes of inflammation.

Inflammation is seen at the site of injury. It is entirely local, although general bodily changes usually take place as well. Inflammation may occur in any tissue of the body. There may be local differences, but by and large, all the body tissues show the same basic changes.

Inflammation is not a disease in itself, it is the reaction of the body to some insult or injury. If there is no injury, there is no inflammation. And if the injurious agent, such as the splinter, is removed, the inflammation fades away. We can then describe inflammation as 'the local and immediate reaction of any body tissue to any insult or injury'.

As with most definitions, there are exceptions. In this case, one big exception to the definition concerns lethal injuries. If the injury kills the patient instantly, then there is no time for inflammation to develop. But if he survives the injury for at least a few hours, then inflammation may be seen.

There are various conditions in which inflammation is one of the main changes. These conditions are given the suffix -*itis*, as in tonsillitis or appendicitis. But inflammation also occurs as a part of many other conditions, the names of which do not end in -*itis*, including such diverse examples as leprosy, burns and sprained ankles.

The five features of inflammation are heat, redness, swelling, pain and loss of function. Thus a sprained ankle feels warm and looks red and swollen compared with the good ankle. It is also painful and may be difficult if not impossible to walk on.

The changes that occur in inflammation can conveniently be considered under five headings—blood flow, capillary permeability, fluid changes, inflammatory cells and tissue cells.

CHANGES IN BLOOD FLOW

In an injured area, the small blood vessels that are not destroyed by the injury show a momentary constriction. This occurs in any injury and will be mentioned again when we come to consider what happens in thrombosis and haemorrhage.

This transient constriction soon passes off, and is followed by an opening up of all the blood vessels in the area. In the normal resting state, some blood vessels are open and some closed, but in inflammation, they are all open wide. The effect of this is to increase the total amount of blood flowing through the injured area (*hyperaemia*).

Another effect is that, although the amount of blood flow is increased to two or three times the usual volume, the actual rate of flow in any one of these vessels decreases—that is, the individual blood cells move more slowly. It is rather like a river in flood, which may break up into several small channels. The total amount of flow is high, but in any one of the small channels, the rate of flow may be sluggish. This happens in an inflamed area, and the sluggishness of the flow may contribute to the formation of thrombi in some of the vessels.

INCREASE OF CAPILLARY PERMEABILITY

Perhaps the most important of all the changes in inflammation is a change in the permeability of the walls of the blood vessels. Normally the walls of small blood vessels allow water and salts and other small molecules to pass in and out with ease. Bigger molecules, such as proteins, cannot normally pass through the vessel walls and they stay in the blood. But in inflammation, large molecules can and do pass out through the vessel walls. Thus water, small molecules and large molecules all pour out through the altered walls of the blood vessels and they form the *inflammatory fluid exudate*. As all the molecules can get out, the composition of this exudate is much the same as that of plasma.

It is traditional to talk of vascular permeability as though it was a passive process, like the enlargement of the holes in a sieve, allowing bigger molecules to get through. There is, however, a good deal of evidence to suggest that the cells lining the small blood vessels are active in this process, that they actively take up molecules from the bloodstream and actively push them out into the tissue spaces.

THE FLUID EXUDATE

In inflammation, the affected part becomes swollen. This is partly due to increased blood volume and partly due to the vast amount of fluid which passes out of the blood vessels into the extracellular tissue spaces as inflammatory oedema. The inflammatory exudate contains many large molecules such as proteins which are normally only found within the blood vessels. These big molecules include fibrinogen, a chemical that is converted into the glue-like substance, fibrin. In the blood vessels fibrin is important in the coagulation of blood to prevent haemorrhage. In inflammation, fibrin is formed outside the blood vessels in the tissues. The fibrin molecules form long strands which act as a framework along which the repair cells can later move. Other big molecules in the exudate are the various nonspecific antibacterial proteins such as properdin, and the specific antibacterial chemicals called antibodies (see Chapter 3).

THE INFLAMMATORY CELLS

About 55 per cent of the blood is fluid, and we have just mentioned what happens to this part of the blood. The other 45 per cent of the blood consists of cells, the red and the white blood cells. A few of the red blood cells may seep out of the blood vessels, but in inflammation it is the white blood cells (leucocytes) that are important.

In inflammation, the white blood cells principally concerned are the *polymorphonuclear leucocytes* (polymorphs or pus cells for short). In inflammation they move out between the cells lining the blood vessel walls and out into the tissue spaces.

They move towards areas of damaged cells, in response to the stimulus provided by a high concentration of cell break-down products in the area. This chemically directed movement is called *chemotaxis*. They proceed to 'eat' the protein and other molecules and particles from broken and damaged cells, a process called *phagocytosis*. They digest this material and break it up into small molecules such as amino acids, which can seep back in the extracellular fluid into the lymphatics and blood vessels and be used again to make protein elsewhere in the body. In summary, the polymorphs show emigration from the blood vessels, movement in one direction due to chemotaxis and then phagocytosis of damaged cell material.

CHANGES IN TISSUE CELLS

The cells of the damaged tissue—whether it be skin, heart muscle, appendix or any other tissue—show changes. Some of them may have been killed or broken. *Necrosis* is the term used for the death of cells. Others may have been damaged but show little immediate change. However, in the succeeding few days, the damage

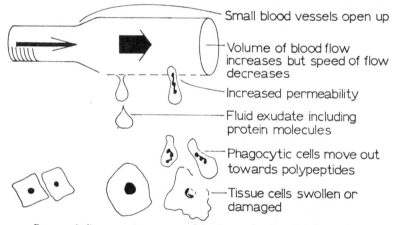

Small blood vessels open up

Volume of blood flow increases but speed of flow decreases

Increased permeability

Fluid exudate including protein molecules

Phagocytic cells move out towards polypeptides

Tissue cells swollen or damaged

FIG. 2-1 A diagrammatic summary of the changes that occur in inflammation

may become obvious. These cells can no longer control the amount of sodium and water they contain. They lose potassium, and take in sodium and water, and can be seen to *swell up* considerably. The cell nucleus shrivels and breaks up and in a short while the whole cell disintegrates and the pieces are phagocytosed. Many more of the tissue cells may also show some degree of swelling, but some of them may recover and survive.

Mechanisms of Inflammation

Many of the experiments that have been done to investigate the process of inflammation have used a small window fitted on to the ear of a rabbit—a rabbit ear chamber. The changes occurring can be seen through the window and studied with a microscope. By this method the effects of inflammation of various nervous and chemical influences have been studied.

From such experiments it appears that nervous reflex action controls the initial transient constriction of the blood vessels by causing constriction of the muscle cells in the vessel walls. The subsequent dilatation of the vessels is also probably due at first to nerve action, but after that it is maintained by the influence of various chemical substances.

Chemical agents are responsible for most of the changes of inflammation. Exactly how they act is still uncertain, but the probable course of events is summarised here.

Within seconds of any damage to the blood vessels in a tissue, the blood platelets stick to the damaged cells lining the vessel wall. They coalesce and release a substance called *histamine*. This chemical acts on the neighbouring vessel-lining cells in some way to increase their permeability. The effect of histamine lasts for perhaps half an hour.

Among the blood proteins, there is a substance called *globulin permeability factor*, which is normally associated with another chemical in the blood which prevents the globulin permeability factor from acting. However, if the blood is diluted in a test-tube, or diluted by seepage out of the blood vessels into the watery tissue fluid as happens in inflammation, the globulin permeability factor becomes active. It breaks down protein molecules derived from injured tissue cells into smaller molecules called *polypeptides*.

The action of the polypeptides on the cells lining the blood vessels is to increase their permeability. Thus the original action of histamine is continued by the polypeptides which result from the activity of the globulin permeability factor. These same polypeptides may also be partly responsible for the chemotactic movements of polymorphs.

GENERALISED BODY CHANGES

In most pathological processes, there are generalised body changes as well as local ones. The generalised changes associated with inflammation include:

    Body temperature increase
    Malaise, poor appetite
    Elevated level of potassium in the serum
    Retention of sodium and water in the body

The protective mechanisms of the body (described in Chapter 3) are sometimes activated in inflammation. There may then be increased numbers of white cells in the blood (leucocytosis), enlargement of the lymph nodes and immune reactions.

EVENTS FOLLOWING INFLAMMATION

What happens following the initial inflammation depends largely on what happens to the cause of the inflammation. If the cause of the inflammation (the splinter or the bacteria) is completely removed or inactivated, then the inflammation fades away (resolution) and the process of repair commences. If the cause of the inflammation persists, then the inflammation persists also, and healing cannot take place. Chronic inflammation occurs if the cause persists for a long time. The injurious agent may then be at the centre of a zone of inflammation, often with repair taking place around the edges of the inflamed area.

Repair

Repair cannot take place in any area until and unless the original injury is completely removed or inactivated. In the case of bacterial infection, repair cannot occur until the bacteria are killed.

Repair is effected by *capillaries* and *fibre-making cells*. The blood vessels of the tissue near the injured area sprout small blind buds which open up to form small capillaries, and these slowly multiply and extend into the injured area. Similarly, the adjacent fibrous tissue cells, and all tissues have some kind of delicate fibrous tissue skeleton, multiply and they actually move into the damaged area where they make new fibres to replace the fine fibrous tissue skeleton that has been destroyed.

The combination of capillaries and fibre-making cells is called *granulation tissue* because it looks granular. The process of conversion of the shapeless mush of dead or damaged tissue into an area with a fibrous tissue skeleton and a blood supply is called *organisation*.

In addition to the fibre-making cells and capillaries, another element is involved in the repair of many tissues and that is the *tissue cells* themselves. In the repair of damaged skin for instance, granulation tissue is seen, but also the skin cells themselves multiply. They undertake regeneration of the damaged skin area but cannot replace damaged skin structures such as hair follicles or sweat glands. The end-result of the repair of a surgical incision is partly fibrous scar tissue and partly regenerated skin. Similar regeneration of the tissue cells occurs in many tissues. Nerve fibres can regenerate but if the cells themselves are damaged, they cannot regenerate. The only other tissue cells that cannot regenerate are muscle cells. In these tissues, there is no regeneration, and it is only granulation tissue that takes part in the repair process, leaving a thick mat of fibrous scar tissue at the site of any injury to nerve cells or muscle.

The measures that promote repair include:

(a) Rest—with avoidance of further stress.
(b) Elevation of the part affected, to assist drainage of the excess tissue fluid.
(c) Drainage of pus.
(d) Moderate heat which speeds up the growth of capillaries and fibre-making cells.
(e) Various chemicals such as antibiotics, to hasten the removal of bacteria.
(f) Diet—especially the correction of deficiencies of essential substances such as Vitamin C.
(g) Other measures—such as attention to fluid balance and cardiac function.

Chronic Inflammation

Chronic inflammation occurs in any situation where the stimulus to inflammation cannot be completely removed or inactivated. In such circumstances the inflammation persists for a long time and attempts at repair also occur, and so chronic inflammation is a combination of inflammation and repair.

In tuberculosis for instance, the bacteria are not readily killed by the defence mechanisms. A tubercle bacillus may persist for years, surrounded by a ring of inflammatory cells, around which is a ring of fibrous tissue. The longer the tubercle bacillus remains, the bigger the lesion may become—with more inflammatory cells and more fibrous tissue, and often with more dead cells at the centre of the lesion due to the action of the bacillus. A lesion like this, composed of concentric rings of inflammatory cells and fibrous tissue, is called a *granuloma*. This is a common form of chronic inflammation and may be seen in many diseases in which bacteria persist in the body, such as tuberculosis, syphilis or leprosy.

Chronic inflammation may also occur if the anatomy of the area is abnormal. For instance, inflammation may become chronic if the blood supply is poor, as in varicose ulcers of the legs. Interference with the normal drainage of tubular structures may have a similar effect, as bacteria or necrotic cells cannot then be removed. In the respiratory tract, for instance, bronchiectasis or a tumour may block the proper drainage of the bronchi. Foreign bodies such as bullets or particles of silica also interfere with the inflammatory response and give rise to chronic inflammation. Fragments of dead bone may have a similar effect.

Another change may be seen adjacent to areas of chronic inflammation, and that is thickening of the lining of the small arteries, a condition called *endarteritis obliterans*. The reason for its occurrence is unknown.

Other examples of chronic inflammation, in which inflammation and repair are seen side by side include rheumatoid arthritis and chronic peptic ulcers. We may note that cortisone and similar agents suppress the formation of granulation tissue in repair. This effect is often helpful in rheumatoid arthritis, but in chronic peptic ulcer the suppression of the repair process may lead to perforation of the wall of the duodenum or stomach.

3 INFECTION AND IMMUNITY

INFECTING ORGANISMS
Entry
Survival within the Body
Disease-producing Mechanisms

THE PROTECTIVE MECHANISMS OF THE HUMAN BODY
Body Surfaces

Non-specific Protective Mechanisms
Chemical Agents
Cellular Non-specific Protective Mechanisms
Interferon

THE SPECIFIC IMMUNE MECHANISMS
Antigens
Lymph Nodes, Liver and Spleen
Antibodies
Specific Immune Cells

Hypersensitivity Reactions
Anaphylactic Shock
Serum Sickness
Allergic Reactions

Various Excesses and Deficiencies of Antibody Production
Hypogammaglobulinaemia
Macroglobulinaemia: Multiple Myelomatosis

Disorders of Cellular Immunity

Auto-immune Diseases
Hashimoto's Disease of the Thyroid
Systemic (or Disseminated) Lupus Erythematosus

THE EFFECTS OF INFECTION—LOCAL AND SYSTEMIC
Local Effects
Inflammation
Pus Formation
Abscess
Granulomas
Infections of Surfaces

Spread of Infection within the Body

Virus Infections

Systemic Effects of Infection

Some Factors which affect the Balance between Pathogenic Organisms and the Human Body

In many parts of the world, the infectious diseases cause more deaths than any other group of diseases. In western countries, the infectious diseases cause fewer deaths, but they still cause more loss of time from school and work than any other disease group.

Infectious diseases are reactions between infecting organisms and patients, and when we consider infectious disease we have to consider both the organisms concerned and the reactions of the patient. It takes two to produce an infectious disease, and the reaction of the patient is just as much a part of the disease process as is the action of the infecting organism.

INFECTING ORGANISMS

We share the surface of the globe with a fantastic number of unseen organisms, most of which are completely harmless and many of which are useful. A few varieties of organisms can, under certain circumstances, cause chemical or other disturbances if they enter our bodies. These ones, the potentially disease-causing ones, are the *pathogenic* organisms.

We cannot avoid coming into contact with pathogenic organisms, and in fact our contacts with them are so common as to be a normal part of our daily lives. A hospital nurse during bed-making may expect to inhale two million or more bacteria every minute, many of which may be pathogenic. We obviously have extremely efficient mechanisms to prevent us from becoming infected. These mechanisms will be described shortly, after some of the characteristics of the pathogenic organisms have been considered.

The organisms capable of producing disease include, in descending order of size, various kinds of worms and flukes such as hook worms, parasites such as malaria, fungi such as thrush (*Candida albicans*), bacteria, mycoplasma and viruses. It is not intended to discuss any of these groups in detail, as the subject is very ably covered in Professor Winner's book, *Microbiology in Patient Care*, in this series. It is, however, necessary to mention some of the ways in which these organisms can cause diseases.

To be able to produce disease, the various infecting organisms have to have:
  (*a*) Some method of entering the human body.
  (*b*) The ability to survive in the internal environment of the human body. This includes resisting the actions of the various protective mechanisms.
  (*c*) Some aspect of their mode of life which disturbs the function of the human body.

ENTRY

Very few organisms can move far enough or fast enough by themselves to enter our bodies. There are very few exceptions to this rule. One is the hook worm, which can penetrate the intact skin of a person's foot, and another is the Leptospira bacteria that can penetrate intact skin from sewer water. But most small organisms cannot move any significant distance. If they enter our bodies, it is because we put them there, by ingesting them, inhaling them or inserting them through a break in the skin during some injury. A few diseases are due to the activities of insects, which insert infecting organisms through the skin when they bite us. For instance, certain mosquitoes transmit malaria and the virus of yellow fever in this way.

SURVIVAL WITHIN THE BODY

The only organisms which can cause disease are those which can survive and multiply in the conditions they encounter in one or more parts of the body. They thrive at a temperature of 37° and in the concentration of salt, the acidity and the other chemical conditions they find. These conditions include the presence of phagocytic cells and antibodies. Many pathogenic organisms possess capsules, tough cell walls or other features which enable them to resist the actions of the body's protective mechanisms.

DISEASE-PRODUCING MECHANISMS

Pathogenic organisms cause diseases by either the chemical or the mechanical disturbances they produce in the patient's body.

The various worms and flukes have complex and sophisticated structures which enable them to utilise *mechanical* factors to their advantage, and the diseases they cause are mainly due to the mechanical disturbances they create. For instance, the filarial worms occupy the lymphatic channels which drain lymph from the tissues, and this leads to a colossal swelling of the soft tissues of the legs or scrotum (*elephantiasis*). The hook worm (*Ankylostoma*) hooks itself on to an intestinal villus, and sucks out blood and tissue fluid. One hook worm may ingest 0·5 ml or more of blood each day, and an infestation of a hundred or more may eventually cause anaemia.

The pathogenic bacteria cause diseases mainly by the action of the *chemicals* they produce. To the bacteria, these chemicals are perhaps the incidental by-products of their existence, but to the human host they are harmful toxins.

Some toxins (*exotoxins*) are secreted by the bacterial cells into their surroundings. The exotoxins are poisonous to human cells in very small amounts, mainly by their chemical action on the enzymes required by human cells for the production of energy from glucose. There are only a few kinds of bacteria which form these powerful exotoxins, namely tetanus, gas gangrene and diphtheria bacteria. The exotoxin-producing bacteria cause disease by secreting exotoxins which affect distant parts of the body although the bacteria stay at the original site of infection. For instance, tetanus bacilli may produce exotoxin at the site of infection in, say, the leg, and a very small amount of the toxin is enough to spread to the central nervous system, and give rise to severe muscle spasms affecting the whole body.

Most bacteria produce *endotoxins* and not the powerful exotoxins. Endotoxins are intracellular chemicals that form part of the structure of the bacterial cells, and they are only released when the bacteria die or are killed and broken up. Endotoxins are generally less powerful poisons than exotoxins, though they all have some harmful effect. In general terms, endotoxins only cause tissue damage when they are concentrated. The endotoxin producers, and these include most bacteria, cause only localised diseases unless they multiply enormously and produce large amounts of endotoxin.

Much less commonly the physical presence of bacteria may be the cause of disease. The exotoxin produced by diphtheria bacilli has already been mentioned, but the bacilli may also cause death by their mechanical presence in the larynx, by combining with inflammatory exudate to form a shaggy membrane which may completely block the airway.

Viruses cause disease by entering human cells, taking charge of their complex control mechanism, and using the cells to produce more virus particles. Normally the structures and cytoplasm of a cell receive instructions as to what chemicals to make from the nucleus. But in a virus-infected cell, the structures in the cytoplasm receive their instructions from the virus, and the instructions are to make more virus material.

By this chemical hijacking, a single virus particle that enters a cell can multiply and be turned into a dozen or more separate virus particles. In some virus diseases, clumps of virus particles called inclusion bodies can be seen down the microscope in the infected cells. Usually the chemistry of the cell is so upset by the takeover that the cell dies, and the virus particles are liberated into the extracellular fluid from which they can infect other cells.

THE PROTECTIVE MECHANISMS OF THE HUMAN BODY

Our numerous daily contacts with pathogenic organisms very seldom lead to infectious disease, and this is entirely due to the efficiency of the various protective mechanisms we possess. These mechanisms act as homeostatic mechanisms, to preserve the internal environment of our bodies undisturbed by foreign agents. The protective mechanisms become more obvious when an infection occurs, for example the 'glands' or lymph nodes in the neck that enlarge in reaction to a throat infection. What is less obvious is that the same protective mechanisms are active all the time, night and day, to prevent the organisms we meet from causing disease.

The various parts of the protective mechanism are most conveniently considered under the headings of body surfaces, non-specific protective mechanisms and specific protective mechanisms. We have also to consider some of the ways in which the protective mechanisms may be deranged and which may themselves be the cause of disease.

Body Surfaces

The skin is the most obvious of the body surfaces, and it has both a mechanical and a chemical barrier to infection. The mechanical barrier of intact skin is its horny outer layer of keratin, which can only be penetrated by a very few organisms, such as the hook worm and Leptospira already mentioned. The chemical barrier to infection is the sweat and the sebaceous secretions, which are supplemented by the chemical activities of the non-pathogenic organisms that live on the skin. These factors tend to clear the skin of any pathogenic organisms that may arrive, by making the chemical conditions inimical to pathogens.

The importance of the skin as a barrier to infection becomes apparent when it is realised how often infections occur when the skin is damaged. Burns, for instance, often become infected, despite the strictest possible precautions.

The outer surfaces between ourselves and the outside world include the respiratory, the alimentary and the urinary tracts. The air passages of the respiratory tract are a large number of branching tubes which are lined by a layer of delicate epithelial cells. This is covered by a thin layer of sticky slime (*mucus*), and it is this slime which traps nearly all the dust particles and bacteria we inhale. The slime is constantly propelled upwards from the chest, by the wafting movement of the cilia of the respiratory epithelial cells, to the larynx, whence it is removed by coughing or swallowing. The slime-trap works well, unless the cilia become paralysed, which happens if the inhaled air is very cold or contains cigarette smoke.

The air sacs of the lungs are all very small, but there are so many of them that together they provide a surface area of 90 square metres for the exchange of oxygen and carbon dioxide. The air sacs are not protected by slime, but by specialised *phagocytic* cells which ingest any particles that arrive, and they transport them to the lymph nodes at the root of the lungs. Some idea of the activity of this system can be gained by examining the lungs of a city-dweller at post-mortem, and noting the large amount of black carbon which has been transported to the lymph nodes.

The alimentary and urinary tracts have somewhat different systems to prevent infection, which will be mentioned later when we come to consider each of these systems separately.

We should mention that under some circumstances, individuals fail to remove pathogenic organisms from one or other of the various body surfaces, although the organisms do not cause any disease. These individuals then are *carriers* of pathogenic organisms. In hospitals, about a quarter of all the doctors and nurses carry pathogenic staphylococci in their noses, perineal skin or elsewhere on their bodies.

Non-specific Protective Mechanisms
If pathogenic organisms penetrate a body surface, they encounter the conditions of the internal environment, and these include the non-specific protective mechanisms, made up of various chemical agents and of phagocytic cells.

CHEMICAL AGENTS
The chemical agents which have been shown to have antibacterial effect against several varieties of bacteria include *lysozyme* and a group of chemicals called *properdins*. Both are present in the blood serum, and lysozyme is also present in various bodily secretions, particularly in tears and nasal secretions. These substances have non-specific antibacterial effects, but it is not known whether or not these effects are important in combating infection, and no method is known of enhancing or of making use of this protective mechanism.

CELLULAR NON-SPECIFIC PROTECTIVE MECHANISMS
Some of the white blood cells, the *polymorphonuclear leucocytes*, are capable of ingesting particles of material that enter our bodies. Polymorphs develop in the bone marrow of the sternum, ribs, vertebrae and pelvis, and are released into the

bloodstream. They circulate in the blood (normally about one polymorph for every thousand red blood cells). In areas of inflammation produced by infection, polymorphs act as they do in any other form of inflammation. They emigrate through the walls of the capillaries, move towards areas of high polypeptide concentration by chemotactic attraction, and then phagocytose bacteria and damaged tissue cells. The ingested material is dissolved by the chemicals the polymorphs contain. In this way, polymorphs dispose of dead cells, bacteria and other particles.

The bone marrow has the task of producing a continuous supply of new polymorphs, as polymorphs can only survive for two or three days outside the bone marrow before they themselves die. In infections, the rate at which new cells are released from the bone marrow is considerably increased, and the number of polymorphs in the blood is increased (*leucocytosis*). In acute appendicitis for instance, the number of white blood cells may increase from the normal range of 5000–11 000 per cubic millimetre to 15 000–25 000 per cubic millimetre. Some of the increased number of polymorphs migrate out through the walls of the capillaries in the appendix, and phagocytose the dead cells and bacteria they encounter there.

Polymorphs are effective in disposing of some kinds of bacteria, and many foreign substances, but not all. For instance, *Pneumococci* have a slimy capsule which effectively prevents phagocytosis. Other organisms such as the bacteria of *gonorrhoea* are phagocytosed, but they are not readily digested within the polymorph and they may even be able to multiply within the polymorph and be released after two or three days when the polymorph itself dies.

The polymorphonuclear leucocytes constitute an effective system for limiting and removing infective organisms and other particles. The system is non-specific in the sense that it operates against not one but many kinds of infecting organisms. However, some organisms cannot be disposed of by this mechanism, and we have other means to cope with them, which will be described shortly.

The main causes of failure of the phagocytic system are the diseases of the blood-forming cells in the bone marrow, *agranulocytosis* and *leukaemia*, which are described in Chapter 9. In agranulocytosis, the bone marrow is incapable of producing adequate numbers of granular white blood cells, principally polymorphs. In leukaemia, the polymorphs produced by the bone marrow are ineffective. In both cases, the individual is very susceptible to infections. These may start as boils or throat infections, with the bacteria multiplying undisturbed and growing in colonies as if they were in bacteriological culture media. The infections may spread and eventually overwhelm the patient.

Kidney transplant patients are in a similar situation, as part of their treatment involves the use of drugs which depress the activity of the bone marrow. Some cancer patients receive similar drugs and they are also very liable to succumb to infections.

INTERFERON

We have already mentioned that in virus infections the viruses invade the cells and take over control of the metabolism of the cell, which is then directed towards making new virus particles. There is in our bodies a mechanism which acts as a non-specific defence against such virus infections, and only against virus infections. This is a chemical substance called *interferon*, which is produced by cells infected by viruses. The interferon produced can diffuse out of one cell and into its uninfected neighbours. In them, interferon in some way alters the control mechanisms of the cell so that viruses can no longer take over the cell metabolism. This is of no benefit to the cells which have already been infected by viruses, and it does not prevent viruses from entering other cells, but it does prevent the viruses from multiplying within the other cells, and this is a considerable advantage in limiting virus infections.

THE SPECIFIC IMMUNE MECHANISMS

A person infected by the measles virus suffers measles, and, as is well known, develops a powerful resistance to any subsequent infection by the same virus. This protection or immunity is specific to the measles virus and it does not protect against infection by any other virus. The development of specific immunity implies that the body in some way recognises, and reacts to, one particular infecting agent.

ANTIGENS

The substances that the specific immune mechanism recognise and react to are called *antigens*. They are mainly proteins or other molecules which have a sufficiently complex structure to be recognised as foreign. Occasionally simpler molecules such as penicillin can act as antigens, if they combine with a body protein, but most simple chemicals do not act as antigens. For instance, sugars may be broken down in the body, or if they are unusual and cannot be broken down they are simply excreted, and they do not provoke an immune reaction. It is only complex foreign substances, mainly protein, and mainly derived from other living organisms, that are recognised as foreign and thus act as antigens. For instance, antigens include various substances formed by bacteria such as exotoxins, and the chemicals of the capsules of bacteria. Other substances recognised as foreign include serum proteins and the surfaces of red blood cells if they are of a foreign blood group.

LYMPH NODES, LIVER AND SPLEEN

Antigenic material, if it enters the body, may reach the extracellular fluid or it may reach the blood. If it enters the extracellular fluid it is carried in the flow along the lymphatic channels to the lymph nodes: if it enters the blood, it is carried in the circulation until it reaches the liver and spleen. The lymphatic vessels in the lymph nodes, and the blood vessels of the liver and spleen are lined by special phagocytic cells called *macrophages* which ingest the foreign material. This uptake of material can be demonstrated by killing and examining an animal such as a mouse after an injection of black carbon particles has been given. The carbon is seen in either the lymph nodes, or the liver and spleen, depending on the precise site of injection.

The macrophages ingest the material, and pass it on to other cells called *lymphocytes*. It is not known for certain whether it is mainly the macrophages or the lymphocytes which recognise the materials as foreign, but it is definitely the lymphocyte cells which react to the foreign material. The lymphocytes can react in two different ways, either by producing *antibodies*, or by multiplying and producing a family of *immune cells* each capable of reacting to any further exposure to the same antigen. When an antigen is detected, cells called B lymphocytes multiply and produce antibodies, and cells called T lymphocytes multiply to produce immune cells.

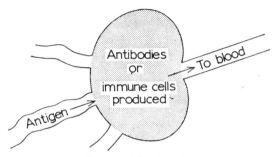

FIG. 3-1 A lymph node

After antigenic material enters the body, there is a delay while the lymphoid cells proliferate and the lymph nodes enlarge. Then, after about seven days, antibodies or immune cells are produced into the blood and they react with the antigen (Figure 3-2).

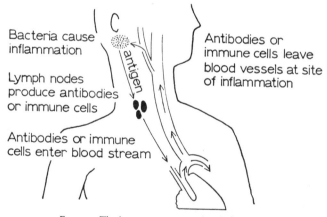

FIG. 3-2 The immune response to an infection

Thereafter the individual is immune to that particular antigen. The immune cells and the state of immunity persist indefinitely. Any second or subsequent exposure to the same antigen produces a much bigger and more rapid response. For instance, the amount of antibody produced in a *secondary response* may be fifty times that of the first or primary response, and it usually takes only a few minutes before antibody appears and only about twenty-four hours until the peak production of antibody is reached.

The specific immunity mechanisms act as the third line of defence, which comes into action if the body surfaces are breached, and if the non-specific chemicals and phagocytes (polymorphs) do not effectively dispose of the foreign material.

ANTIBODIES

The production of antibodies occurs mainly in the lymph nodes and the spleen. The B lymphocytes which produce antibodies change their appearance, and they are then given the name *plasma cells*, as they were first noticed in blood plasma. The antibody they produce is a chemical which is formed in such a way that it combines with one particular antigen and only one. For instance, the antibody that is formed in lobar pneumonia dissolves the antigen in the capsules of the infecting pneumococci, but only the capsules of that strain of pneumococcus. Dissolving the capsule exposes the bacteria, which can then be phagocytosed by polymorphs. Different antibodies are named according to their main effect. *Antitoxins*, for instance, are antibodies that combine with and neutralise bacterial toxins.

The antibodies produced by the plasma cells are released into the blood stream. Antibodies are proteins and they form the group of proteins in the blood serum known as *gamma globulins*. Like other proteins, they circulate in the blood and can only enter the tissues at places where inflammation has made the walls of the capillaries more permeable than normal. This means that antibodies are not scattered throughout the whole body, but are only present in the bloodstream and at sites of tissue damage and inflammation, and they are thus restricted to the sites where they are most likely to be needed.

SPECIFIC IMMUNE CELLS

In some cases, the lymph nodes react not by producing chemical antibodies but by producing a family of cells which are capable of dealing with a particular antigen. This happens particularly when the antigen is fixed to the tissues and is not free to circulate in the body. For instance, in Contact Dermatitis, some chemical may get on to and irritate the skin and act as an antigen. The local lymph nodes then react by producing a family of *immune cells* which, like chemical antibodies, pass into the circulating blood and eventually out of the blood vessels in the inflamed area of the skin. The mechanism by which these immune cells dispose of the antigen is not fully known, but it is certain that these cells carry chemical substances which can encourage phagocytic cells to congregrate around the antigen and phagocytose it. This specific cellular mechanism of immunity is important in the defence reactions against some bacteria, particularly tuberculosis, and against many viruses. The same mechanism is involved in the rejection of foreign tissues, such as transplanted kidneys, and attempts must then be made to suppress the activities of these specific immune cells.

Hypersensitivity Reactions

In many cases the body's reaction to antigen is a life-saving defence mechanism. In some cases, however, the reaction itself may be more trouble than the antigen.

In some individuals, for instance, the reaction to innocuous pollens may be excessive and give rise to hay fever. This is a hypersensitivity reaction.

The hypersensitivity reactions include anaphylactic shock, atopic reactions and serum sickness; in all of which antibodies react in different ways with antigen.

ANAPHYLACTIC SHOCK

In man, an initial sensitising exposure to an antigenic substance such as penicillin may lead to the development of antibodies which become attached to certain histamine-containing cells. After a second exposure (the *shocking* dose), the antigen rapidly comes in contact with the pre-existing antibody on the cell surfaces, and the reaction between antigen and antibody causes the cells to release their histamine. The histamine causes the muscle in the walls of the bronchioles to contract smartly, causing acute respiratory distress, like asthma. Similar chemical substances released from other antibody-coated cells may cause a redness and itching of the skin, and increase of capillary permeability leading to generalised oedema (Figure 3-3).

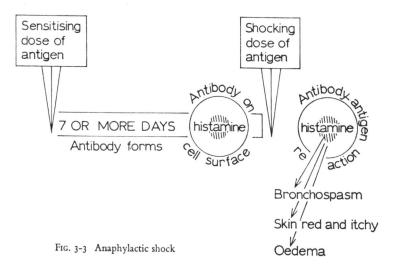

Fig. 3-3 Anaphylactic shock

SERUM SICKNESS

This is another form of antigen-antibody reaction. In this case, a single dose of antigen is enough to produce the changes seen, though a relatively large dose is necessary. The single dose of material such as 'foreign' serum leads to the formation of antibodies after about a week. The antibodies combine with the antigen which remains in the blood, and produces aggregates of antigen-antibody complex which tend to clog the smaller blood vessels. The effects are most marked in the kidneys, where the complexes become trapped in the capillaries of the glomeruli and cause a from of glomerulonephritis. Similar changes elsewhere may give rise to myocarditis in the heart muscle, urticaria in the skin and pain in the joints (Figure 3-4).

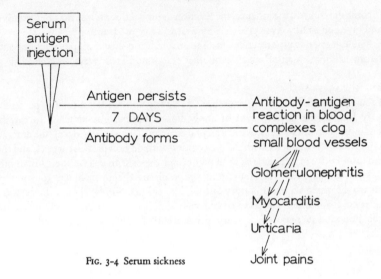

FIG. 3-4 Serum sickness

ALLERGIC REACTIONS

Some unfortunate individuals develop antibodies in reaction to traces of foreign protein in certain foods, drugs, dusts and pollens. Some of the affected individuals have a family history of similar complaints. The antibodies formed become attached to the surfaces of cells, often in the skin or in the lining of the respiratory tract. Any subsequent exposure to the same antigens produces an antigen–antibody reaction on the surface of the cells and produces hay fever or eczema, or one of the varieties of asthma (Figure 3-5).

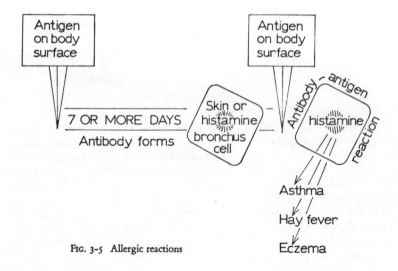

FIG. 3-5 Allergic reactions

Various Excesses and Deficiencies of Antibody Production

HYPOGAMMAGLOBULINAEMIA

A low level of antibodies in the blood is called *hypogammaglobulinaemia*. It is due to deficient antibody production, as a result of some abnormality in the lymphoid tissues. Occasionally, in a child, this is due to a faulty development of the lymph nodes. The condition also occasionally develops in patients with tumours of the lymphoid tissues, such as *lymphosarcoma* or *chronic lymphoid leukaemia*. Whether the condition is congenital or is acquired later, the patients are very liable to develop infections, especially infections caused by Staphylococci, Streptococci and Pneumococci.

MACROGLOBULINAEMIA: MULTIPLE MYELOMATOSIS

In macroglobulinaemia, there is an abnormal proliferation of the antibody-forming cells, the cause of which is unknown. In the blood there are large amounts of abnormal antibody molecules, joined together to form large macroglobulins from which the disease gets its name. The condition is uncommon. It affects men over 50, and they suffer from weight loss and eventually die due to an abnormal susceptibility to infections.

Multiple myelomatosis is less rare, though it is still not common. It affects men and women equally, and they are almost exclusively between the ages of 55 and 65. Multiple myelomatosis is a malignant condition of the antibody-forming cells, which proliferate to form tumorous masses in the marrow of the bones, especially the skull, the vertebrae, pelvis and ribs. The tumour cells form enormous quantities of partly-formed antibody molecules. These abnormal proteins can be detected in the blood, and also in the urine (as Bence-Jones protein). The abnormal antibody molecules in the blood may contribute to *amyloidosis*, a condition which may complicate multiple myelomatosis (Chapter 6).

Disorders of Cellular Immunity

The lymph nodes are principally concerned in cellular immunity. We might therefore expect that patients with tumours originating in the lymph nodes would show abnormalities of the specific cellular immunity mechanism, and indeed they often do. In some cases there is an excessive production of lymphocytes. These may infiltrate the body tissues and they may also appear in the blood, as lymphocytic leukaemia. In some cases, a defect of immune function can also be demonstrated. In Hodgkin's disease for instance, some patients show little or no lymphocytic reaction to intradermal injections of tuberculo-protein, despite previous exposure to tuberculosis. This test is of some practical importance as it demonstrates a defect in specific cellular immunity which renders these patients particularly liable to infection by such agents as viruses and fungi, and such infections are not infrequently fatal.

Auto-immune Diseases

Our immune mechanisms are able to distinguish between the chemicals of our own bodies and any 'foreign' chemicals, such as bacterial substances. Normally this distinction between 'self' and 'not self' chemicals is rapidly and accurately made. The 'not self' chemicals are then treated as 'foreign' antigens and are destroyed.

Very occasionally the system fails, and the immune mechanisms react against one or more of the constituents of our own bodies. This may be due to some subtle change in one of the 'self' constituents of the body, or to some change in the immune mechanism which somehow fails to recognise a 'self' chemical. Whatever the cause, the result is one of the auto-immune diseases.

These diseases are uncommon, and we do not know the full story about any of them, but they are important enough to warrant a brief account of some of their features. The auto-immune diseases include Hashimoto's disease of the thyroid, Systemic Lupus Erythematosus, Auto-immune Haemolytic Anaemia, probably Idiopathic Thrombocytopenic Purpura and probably Rheumatoid Arthritis. There are other diseases of unknown cause which may also have an auto-immune basis, such as Polyarteritis Nodosa, Glomerulonephritis and Rheumatic Fever. Perhaps we can take two of the conditions from this formidable list and use them as examples.

HASHIMOTO'S DISEASE OF THE THYROID

It is principally the cellular side of the specific immunity mechanism that is responsible for Hashimoto's disease, although in many cases antibody production is also present. In some other auto-immune diseases such as auto-immune haemolytic anaemia, antibody production is the principal factor, and cellular immunity probably plays little part.

In Hashimoto's disease, the thyroid gland becomes packed with large numbers of lymphocytes, and this is associated with gradual destruction of the gland tissue. Eventually, the gland is reduced to a fibrous relic, and the resulting deficiency of thyroid hormone production is seen as myxoedema. Antibodies against some of the proteins of thyroid tissue are present in the blood of many of the patients with this condition, but the quantity of such antibodies bears little relationship to the severity of the gland destruction, and it is probably the cellular immune reaction which is the main process in this disease. The disease almost exclusively affects middle-aged women.

SYSTEMIC (OR DISSEMINATED) LUPUS ERYTHEMATOSUS (S.L.E.)

Systemic Lupus Erythematosus is almost certainly an auto-immune disease due to the presence of abnormal antibodies in the blood. These antibodies react with and damage cell nuclei. The nuclei of white blood cells from a normal person are damaged if they are incubated with the serum of a patient with Systemic Lupus Erythematosus. This is the basis of the L.E. test.

Systemic Lupus Erythematosus is a diffuse disorder affecting many parts of the body. It mainly occurs in young women. It has a slow onset with mild fever, pain moving from joint to joint and a rash over the bridge of the nose, usually in the shape of a butterfly. Blood vessel changes occur, which can be seen in the eyes as retinal exudates and which in the kidney cause proteinuria. The diffuse nature of the disease can be appreciated from the occurrence sometimes of pleural effusions, pericarditis or endocarditis. The disease usually runs a prolonged up-and-down course with remissions and is not usually fatal, but occasionally death occurs due to renal failure.

THE EFFECTS OF INFECTION—LOCAL AND SYSTEMIC

We will close this chapter with a brief account of some of the possible effects, both local and systemic, of the reaction between an infecting organism and the infected patient.

Local Effects

INFLAMMATION

All pathogenic bacteria cause some degree of local tissue damage, and some degree of localised inflammation is always present, The stimulus to inflammation lasts for as long as the bacteria continue to exist.

PUS FORMATION (Suppuration)

Pus formation is nearly always due to bacterial infection. The bacteria most commonly responsible are the ones with a high multiplication rate, which can achieve a considerable degree of local tissue destruction by endotoxin accumulation, before the inflammatory response, phagocytosis and the specific immunity mechanisms can dispose of the organisms. Pus is the thick, yellow or greenish fluid that results from the local destruction of tissue cells. The constituents of pus in an infection are:

Tissue cells—dead or damaged.
Infecting organisms such as bacteria—living or dead.
Polymorphs and/or lymphocytes—living or dead.
Various chemicals of the inflammatory exudate—such as antibodies, fibrin and the constituents of serum.

ABSCESS

An abscess is a cavity formed by local tissue destruction and filled with pus. If the bacteria can be killed, small abscesses can heal by absorption of the tissue debris and by fibrosis to close the cavity. In larger abscesses, the quantity of semi-fluid debris to be disposed of may be more than the polymorphs can readily accomplish, and continuing tissue damage may occur due to toxins. The further tissue damage usually affects the nearest soft tissues, and the abscess is then said to 'point' or 'track'. To prevent such further tissue damage, surgeons prefer to drain large abscesses.

A 'cold abscess' is a tuberculous abscess. It is so called because its wall is formed mainly of fibrous tissue and it shows little surrounding inflammation.

GRANULOMAS

In other bacterial infections, principally the chronic infections such as tuberculosis, the tissue damage is less severe as the organisms only multiply slowly and they produce little endotoxin. The main feature of such organisms is their capacity to survive all the efforts of the protective mechanisms of the body to dispose of them. In these cases, each small group of organisms produces a small area of necrosis, which becomes surrounded by a zone of inflammation, and around which a thick layer of granulation and fibrous tissue develops. Over the years, the organisms may slowly multiply and cause further tissue necrosis, and the combination of the inflammation and repair processes may produce a thicker and thicker fibrous wall to the lesion.

INFECTIONS OF SURFACES

Infections frequently involve a body surface without entering the tissues. Examples of this include the dysenteries and cholera which affect the intestinal surface. Such infections differ from tissue infections as the organisms are not readily localised and they may be scattered over a wide area of the surface. As a result, a large area may become inflamed. Another feature of such infection is that there may be a tremendous out-pouring of inflammatory cells and inflammatory exudate, to make up for the fact that much of the exudate may be dissipated or lost to the outside world.

Spread of Infection within the Body

The capacity for an infecting organism to produce disease may be adequately balanced by the protective mechanisms of the patient, and in this case the organisms may localise and can often be disposed of. On the other hand, if the organisms can multiply more rapidly than the patient can mobilise the various components of the protective mechanism, the organisms are likely to spread.

Organisms may spread within the infected tissue, as erysipelas does in the skin, or through tissue spaces such as the pleural cavities or the peritoneum. Spread of infecting organisms along the lymphatic channels is common, and causes an inflammation of the lymphatics called *lymphangitis*. This may be seen as a red streak up the forearm following some infections of the hand. The phagocytic cells in the lymph nodes act as traps for the infecting organisms, which usually, but not always are successful in preventing further spread of the organisms via the lymphatic channels. Occasionally, infecting organisms become trapped in a lymph node, but cannot be effectively disposed of, and then they may be the cause of an abscess forming in the lymph node.

Organisms may enter a blood vessel and be spread by the bloodstream. For instance, when we have a tooth extracted, we all have a transient bacteraemia, but the organisms are usually phagocytosed within a few minutes, either by the polymorphs in the blood or by the phagocytic cells in the liver and spleen.

Occasionally, such organisms are not rapidly removed, and they may give rise to widespread metastatic abscesses in different organs of the body. For instance, an abscess in the lung may disseminate organisms via the bloodstream and give rise to metastatic abscesses in the brain and elsewhere, in much the same way as a lung tumour may give rise to metastatic tumour deposits in the brain and elsewhere.

The name *septicaemia* is used when bacteria enter the blood, and flourish and multiply within the bloodstream itself. This is obviously an extremely serious state of affairs, as it indicates that the protective mechanisms of the body have been overwhelmed. The organisms concerned may not produce powerful toxins, but there are many of them and they are widespread. The muscle cells in the walls of the arterioles are damaged and can no longer constrict, and the loss of peripheral vasoconstriction causes severe endotoxic shock and death.

Virus Infections

Viruses cause the destruction of the individual cells infected, and these are usually the cells of a body surface in the first instance, such as the skin and mucosal covering of the eyes, nose and mouth in measles. Virus infections may lead to:

(a) Complete recovery with replacement of the surface cells damaged.

(b) Spread of virus to lymph nodes, bloodstream and thence to the susceptible cells anywhere in the body, such as the nerve cells in the spinal cord in poliomyelitis.

(c) Secondary infection by bacteria. This is particularly common in the respiratory tract.

Systemic Effects of Infection

All pathological processes have local effects and general bodily effects, and infection is no exception. As already mentioned, infection is always accompanied by some degree of inflammation, and the systemic changes in inflammation include temperature, malaise, increased adrenal steroid hormones, retention of sodium, elevated blood potassium and increased protein breakdown (Chapter 2).

In infection, the reaction of the protective mechanisms produces other prominent changes including an increased number of polymorphs in the blood (leucocytosis), enlargement of lymph nodes and increased antibody levels in the blood. This latter is probably the cause of the increased erythrocyte sedimentation rate (E.S.R.).

Another prominent feature of many bacterial infections is fever, particularly in children and rather less markedly in old people. Fever is not just the result of increased heat production by the cells, as such an increase of heat production occurs in most athletic pursuits and yet, by sweating, the athlete can keep his body temperature remarkably constant. The fever is the result of the action of endotoxic substances called *pyrogens*, produced by bacteria and acting on the temperature-controlling mechanism of the brain. The onset of fever is usually accompanied by a complaint of feeling cold, and shivering, which is muscular activity, which increases the heat production. Excessive sweating often accompanies the end of a fever, and the sweating is the mechanism by which the body temperature is lowered. One of the actions of aspirins is to reduce a raised body temperature in this way.

Bacterial infections are not the only causes of temperature increase (*pyrexia*). Any inflammatory process may be accompanied by some degree of pyrexia. Heat stroke, with excessive sodium loss usually shows marked pyrexia. Pyrexia may also follow severe tissue damage, such as a *myocardial infarct*. Tissue damage may also account for the curious fluctuating pyrexia commonly seen in Hodgkin's disease of the lymphoid tissues.

One other systemic change occurring in some bacterial infections (tetanus, diphtheria and gas gangrene) is the action of the exotoxins on different body tissues, as mentioned earlier in this chapter.

Some Factors which affect the Balance between Pathogenic Organisms and the Human Body

The defence mechanisms of the body do not work effectively in dead or damaged tissues. In such areas, bacteria may multiply freely. Other factors which favour bacterial infection are the presence of pre-existing disease, disorders of the protective mechanisms or chemical deficiencies.

(1) *Local Tissue Damage*—Tissue damage is obvious and visible when caused by surgical incisions or accidental laceration of the skin. Other instances include infection of tissues deprived of their blood supply, e.g. surgical sutures too tight, infections of toes and feet in patients with severe arterial disease, infections of extremities after frostbite. Local tissue damage includes damage by particles such as silica in the lung, which facilitate tuberculous infection.

(2) *Pre-existing Diseases*—Patients with diseases in which the general metabolism of all the body cells is upset, such as diabetes and chronic renal failure, are very liable to infection.

(3) *Disturbances of the Protective Mechanisms*—Leukaemias, tumours of the lymph nodes and the like have been mentioned earlier in this chapter. We can remind ourselves that the actions of the immune mechanisms can sometimes be enhanced for the patient's benefit, either by giving antibodies, such as Anti-Tetanus Serum (ATS) or by stimulating increased antibody production, such as by Tetanus Toxoid injection (TT), or by stimulating cellular immunity, such as by BCG (Bacillus Calmette-Guérin) to stimulate cellular immunity to tuberculosis bacilli.

(4) *Non-specific Chemical Deficiencies*—Deficiencies of vitamin A and vitamin C both reduce the general level of resistance to infection, and so does starvation.

(5) *Antibiotics and Similar Drugs*—We can alter the internal environment marvellously for the patient's benefit, provided we know what organism is present, what antibiotic it is sensitive to and that the organism is not isolated from the antibiotic by a wall of pus or fibrosis. Note that antibiotics can occasionally alter the balance the other way, e.g. Tetracycline may kill most of the organisms normally resident in the gut, and allow pathogenic organisms to flourish there, such as resistant Staphylococci.

(6) *Rest*—Movement of the body may assist the spread of infecting organisms. General stresses and strains are also thought to hinder healing, perhaps by increasing the secretion of the adrenal steroid hormones which tend to suppress the inflammatory reaction and the production of lymphocytes which form the specific cellular immunity mechanism.

4 VARIOUS CIRCULATORY DISTURBANCES

Chronic Venous Congestion

Oedema

Haemorrhage
Vascular Damage
Platelet and Coagulation Factor Deficiencies

Shock

Thrombosis

Embolism

Ischaemia
Gangrene

Chronic Venous Congestion

Chronic venous congestion means a sluggish flow of blood round the body. It may be due to diseases of the heart muscle, diseases of the heart valves or diseases of the lungs. Diseases of the heart muscle are the commonest causes of chronic venous congestion. When either the heart muscle or the heart valves are affected, the pumping action of the heart is impaired, and this is referred to as congestive cardiac failure. The lung diseases which cause chronic venous congestion are emphysema and fibrosis. In these diseases, the blood vessels in the lungs are damaged and the amount of blood that can flow through the lungs and back to the heart is severely reduced (Figure 4-1).

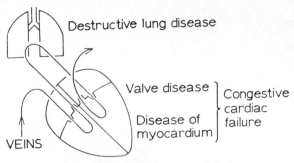

FIG. 4-1   Causes of chronic venous congestion

Whether the cause be heart disease or destructive lung disease, the result is a reduced movement of blood around the body. This affects all the organs and tissues of the body, but it is most noticeable in the veins. The flow in the veins is never very rapid, and even a slight reduction may cause venous congestion.

So chronic venous congestion means congestion of the veins, but it also means a sluggish blood flow and the effects thereof on all parts of the body.

In the lungs, the poor blood flow means that only a small amount of blood becomes oxygenated, and this causes shortness of breath (*dyspnoea*), and it may also cause oedema of the lungs. In the systemic circulation, the neck veins may be distended with blood, and there may be oedema of the lower parts of the body.

Chronic venous congestion has serious effects on the internal organs, including the liver. The normal liver is of an even brown colour, but in chronic venous congestion the liver cells cannot properly perform their functions and in particular cannot deal with fat. Fat accumulates and makes the liver cells appear pale and greasy. At the same time, the small veins draining the liver are congested, and show as small dark spots. These dark spots scattered through the pale liver tissue give it the name of 'nutmeg liver'. If this state of affairs persists for long enough, some of the liver cells die and are replaced by fibrous scar tissue, and this condition is called *cardiac cirrhosis*.

The kidneys may be similarly affected. Their function may also be disturbed and they may be capable of producing only a small quantity of urine (*oliguria*), and the urine may contain some protein.

The liver and kidneys have been mentioned as examples of the effects of chronic venous congestion. All the other organs are similarly affected, and none is exempt.

Oedema

Normally the amount of water that passes out of the blood vessels into the tissue spaces is limited by two factors. One is that protein molecules exert an attraction on water molecules. The other is that protein molecules cannot normally escape from the blood vessels. Thus protein molecules tend to hold water molecules within the blood vessels.

When this system is upset, an excess of water collects in the spaces between the cells, and this constitutes oedema. An oedematous tissue is waterlogged. It feels soggy, and in oedematous skin a doughy pit can be produced by pressing with a finger.

We have already mentioned that in inflammation, an increase of capillary wall permeability allows protein molecules to escape into the tissues. Water molecules move out with the protein molecules into the tissues, and inflammation is an important cause of oedema. The oedema it causes is local, it only occurs in the inflamed area.

Oedema also occurs locally if there is a blockage, such as a thrombus, in a vein draining the blood from a particular area. In this case, the force of attraction on the water molecules by protein molecules is not as strong as the force of the increased pressure due to the blocked vein. The water molecules are virtually pushed out through the walls of the capillaries by the pressure.

Normally the lymphatic channels drain away some of the tissue fluid. Local oedema may occur if these lymphatic channels are blocked, for instance, by cancer cells in some cases of breast cancer. More dramatic is the massive oedema of the legs and scrotum which occurs if the lymphatic channels become blocked by the tiny filarial worms of elephantiasis.

We have mentioned three causes of local oedema, but oedema may also be generalised and affect the whole body. In such cases, the excess tissue fluid is most obvious in the lowest soft part of the body; that is in the ankles, or, in patients confined to bed, in the skin over the sacrum. In generalised oedema, fluid may also collect in the lungs ((*pulmonary oedema*) or in any of the serous sacs. The fluid may be in the pleural spaces (*hydrothorax*), the peritoneum (*ascites*) or less commonly in the pericardium (*hydropericardium*).

The commonest cause of generalised oedema is chronic venous congestion. The oedema is presumably due to the effect of 'back pressure' on the veins throughout the body that occurs in chronic venous congestion.

Protein deficiency, due to starvation, malabsorption or loss of protein in the urine in kidney disease, also causes generalised oedema. In this case, the water molecules escape into the tissues because there is insufficient protein to hold them in the blood vessels.

Sodium retention, due to hormone disorders, is a third cause of generalised oedema, and it is also found frequently in pregnancy.

TABLE 4-1 *Causes of oedema*

Local	General
Inflammation	Chronic venous congestion
Thrombosis of vein	Sodium retention
Lymphatic blockage	Protein deficiency
(e.g. by cancer cells	(Starvation, malabsorption
or filariasis)	or kidney disease)

The presence of an excess of tissue fluid is harmful to the cells as it impairs their nutrition. However, the significance of oedema is that it indicates that some serious disease state must be present to cause it.

Pulmonary oedema has a significance of its own, as it may kill the patient. It starts with a dry irritant cough. Later, fine bubbling sounds called *crepitations* may be heard at the bottom of the lungs, due to fluid in the smaller bronchi. In more severe pulmonary oedema, watery fluid collects in the air spaces at the bottom of the lungs, and the lungs may gradually fill up with fluid until no air exchange is possible, and death occurs.

Haemorrhage

VASCULAR DAMAGE

Most cases of haemorrhage are due to physical injury to fairly large blood vessels and require little comment. In these cases, the normal process of thrombus formation is not adequate to control the escape of blood.

Haemorrhage may also occur from smaller blood vessels if the cells that form the walls of these vessels are damaged chemically by the action of bacterial toxins in septicaemia or acute infections. Numerous small haemorrhages may also occur in some cases of chronic renal failure (*uraemia*) and these may be due to the effect of the severe biochemical changes on the same cells in the walls of the small blood vessels. Small *petechial* haemorrhages may then be seen in the skin and the mucous membranes of the mouth. Further unseen haemorrhages may occur in the internal organs.

Similar changes are seen in Henoch-Schönlein purpura. These are probably also due to damage to the walls of the small blood vessels, but the precise cause is unknown. The disease may have an allergic basis, or it may perhaps be an auto-immune disease.

PLATELET AND COAGULATION FACTOR DEFICIENCIES

We are continually doing minor damage to our blood vessels, such as when we are thrown against the metalwork of a bus or cut ourselves while shaving. Most of us are capable of forming a small thrombus at the site of injury which prevents haemorrhage from the damaged vessel. This is the normal reaction to an injury to a blood vessel. It involves three changes which take place in sequence (Figure 4-2).

(1) The muscle cells in the walls of the injured vessel contract, reducing the blood flow.

(2) The blood platelets stick to the cells which line the injured blood vessel, and form a platelet plug.

(3) A series of chemical reactions takes place in the blood, one after another. The last of these is the conversion of the soluble substance fibrinogen, a protein found in the blood or in inflammatory exudate, into strands of insoluble fibrin. The fibrin strands form a rough network, like a beaver's dam across a stream. Red and white blood cells and platelets become trapped in the network and the thrombus is complete. The conversion of fibrinogen into fibrin can only take place if the various substances needed for the preceding reactions are present in normal quantities.

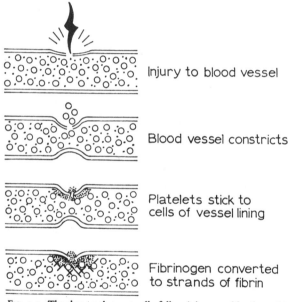

Injury to blood vessel

Blood vessel constricts

Platelets stick to cells of vessel lining

Fibrinogen converted to strands of fibrin

FIG. 4-2 The changes that normally follow injury to a blood vessel

Let us consider each of these three stages in turn.

(1) Contraction of the walls of the vessels reduces the blood flow. Without this reduction, the blood platelets would be swept away as soon as they started to form a plug. It is for this reason that other methods of reducing the local blood flow are often helpful. For instance, the gentle pressure of a thumb for a minute or two over the bleeding site is often effective in allowing a thrombus to form in a small blood vessel, such as may be damaged during shaving. A pad, such as a clean handkerchief, can be used to provide pressure over a bleeding site if larger blood vessels are damaged.

(2) The platelet plug can only be formed if there is an adequate supply of platelets. Blood platelets (thrombocytes) are small particles which are made, like blood

cells, in the bone marrow. Diseases of the bone marrow may reduce platelet production and then numerous small haemorrhages (purpura) may occur (*thrombocytopenic purpura*).

(3) The chemicals which take part in the reactions leading to fibrin formation include fibrinogen, prothrombin, antihaemophilic globulin and Christmas factor. A deficiency of any one of these causes poor thrombus formation, and may be seen either as numerous small haemorrhages, or as persistent oozing of blood from some small blood vessel which may go on for days and days.

Fibrinogen deficiency (*Hypofibrinogenaemia*) may occur if the fibrinogen in the blood is used up. This may happen if some of the chemicals involved in the earlier stages of the clotting mechanism are released into the blood and the occasions when this is most likely to occur are as a complication of pregnancy in accidental haemorrhage or amniotic fluid embolism, or in some bypass operations for heart or lung surgery. In these cases, the fibrinogen is turned into fibrin in the bloodstream, and this uses up all the available fibrinogen. The deficiency of fibrinogen can be made good by fibrinogen transfusions, and this may be necessary to prevent widespread haemorrhages. Fibrinogen is made in the liver and hypofibrinogenaemia may sometimes be seen in patients with severe liver disease.

Prothrombin is made in the liver from vitamin K. Deficiencies of prothrombin may occur in malabsorption (vitamin K is fat-soluble) or in liver disease. Anticoagulant drugs of the *dicoumarol* type are used to prevent excessive thrombus formation. They inhibit the production of prothrombin, and over-enthusiastic use of such anticoagulants sometimes causes purpuric haemorrhages or oozing.

Antihaemophilic globulin is another of the chemicals required for adequate conversion of fibrinogen to fibrin. Most of us have an adequate supply of antihaemophilic globulin, but a small number of males have a deficient production and they suffer from *Haemophilia*. It is a congenital abnormality which is inherited as a sex-linked recessive disease. Females carry the defective gene without any sign of the disease, but all their sons have haemophilia. In haemophilia, any injury is liable to be followed by persistent oozing which may go on and on for days or weeks. Bleeding into a joint cavity such as the knee joint commonly occurs, and tooth extractions may be followed by persistent and severe haemorrhage. Fresh blood or concentrated anti-haemophilic globulin from normal people may be necessary to correct the deficiency and enable normal thrombosis to occur.

Christmas factor deficiency is very similar to Haemophilia, but less common. It also is inherited as a sex-linked recessive characteristic.

In summary, haemorrhage may be due to injury, to toxic damage to the cells in the walls of the small blood vessels in septicaemia and the like, to deficiencies in platelets (thrombocytopenic purpura) or to deficiencies of one of the coagulation factors. If blood coagulation is defective it is sometimes necessary to resort to sophisticated tests to determine which of the coagulation factors may be responsible.

Shock

The principal change in shock is a reduction of the arterial blood pressure. The normal pressure of the blood in the arteries depends on:

(*a*) The pressure provided by the pumping action of the heart, at one end of the arterial tree.

(*b*) The volume of blood within the arteries.

(*c*) The resistance at the other end of the tree provided by the arterioles. The arterioles are numerous small channels, each of which has muscle cells in its wall by means of which the arteriole can contract. This contraction narrows the vessel, restricts the flow of blood out of the arterial tree and raises the blood pressure.

If the pumping action of the heart fails, or the volume of blood in the arteries is reduced, or the arterioles become excessively dilated, then the blood pressure falls, and the patient is in a state of shock (Figure 4-3). He is pale and cold, and has a

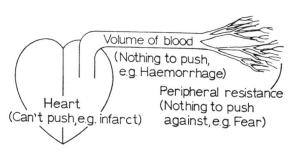

FIG. 4-3 Shock

bluish skin, low blood pressure and a thin feeble rapid pulse. He may be thirsty and have little or no output of urine, and there may be a concentration of the blood cells due to loss of the fluid part of the blood into the tissues.

By far the commonest cause of central or cardiac shock is *myocardial infarction*. It may also occur in massive pulmonary embolism and other less common catastrophes which may damage the pumping mechanism of the heart, such as cardiac tamponade.

The term *oligaemic* shock covers various conditions in which the blood pressure is reduced by a reduction in the blood volume. It occurs in severe haemorrhage, in burns (largely due to the large amount of fluid lost from the body through the burnt skin) and in severe dehydrating conditions such as cholera.

Anaphylactic shock in man does not really fit into any of our three categories of shock, but perhaps it can be mentioned with oligaemic shock. In anaphylaxis, the most marked effect is severe asthma-like bronchospasm. There may also be a severe fall of blood pressure, perhaps due to a widespread increase of capillary permeability. This causes a marked reduction of blood volume as fluid leaves the blood vessels and enters the tissue and rapidly gives rise to generalised oedema.

An example of shock due to arteriolar dilatation is *bacteraemic* or *endotoxic* shock. In this case, the cells forming the walls of the small blood vessels are damaged by the chemical effects of bacterial toxins in the blood. The small blood vessels lose their power to constrict, and they all open up together. The fall in blood pressure that this produces may be fatal.

A confusing feature of shock is that nervous stimuli can produce some of its changes, such as dilatation of the arterioles and a drop in blood pressure. This happens when someone faints. The nervous stimuli include fear, anxiety and pain or even the anticipation of pain. Some people, even brave people, faint at the sight of an injection needle due to the dilatation of the arterioles produced by nervous stimuli. After lying down for a few minutes, the neurogenic shock or fainting passes off.

However, such an incident of neurogenic shock may complicate the picture in other kinds of shock. For example, a man suffering a myocardial infarct may faint with the pain and anxiety associated with the infarct. When the pain passes off, he may regain consciousness and appear normal for a short while, with a more or less normal blood pressure. A little later, the effect of the infarct on the myocardium becomes apparent and the blood pressure falls again, this time more severely, due to cardiac shock.

When the blood pressure falls from any cause, the blood flow around the body is poor, and all the functions of the body suffer. If the blood flow is not restored, the cells lining the blood capillaries may be so damaged that they allow protein and water molecules to stream out into the tissues. This is called *irreversible shock*, because at this stage, the control of the internal environment of the tissue cells has completely collapsed, and only death can follow.

In some heart and lung operations, a heart-lung apparatus is used to bypass and take over the functions of the heart and lungs. Occasionally during such operations the blood pressure may accidentally fall. In these cases the result is not irreversible shock, as the circulation is maintained mechanically, but severe damage is done to some tissue cells. The cells most sensitive are those of the brain and the kidney tubules, and such damage results in impaired mental faculties or acute tubular necrosis of the kidneys, which is itself sometimes fatal.

Thrombosis

Thrombus formation only constitutes a disease process when it occurs at the wrong time or place. The thrombi that we form after injuries to prevent bleeding are entirely normal.

The three important factors in the abnormal formation of thrombi are disease of the lining of a blood vessel, a reduced rate of blood flow and increased stickiness of the blood platelets (Figure 4-4). The lining of a blood vessel may be altered by the spread of nearby infection or by the degenerative changes of atherosclerosis (Chapter 7).

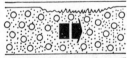 Abnormal vessel wall
Slow blood flow
Sticky platelets

FIG. 4-4 Factors which promote thrombus formation

A reduced rate of blood flow occurs in the small blood vessels in an area of inflammation, and this often leads to thrombosis. A reduced flow also occurs in the veins in chronic venous congestion, and in the veins of patients lying in bed. A reduced flow can even occur in the heart and lead to thrombosis, if there are abnormal contraction waves (atrial fibrillation). This occurs sometimes in the left atrium, where a pool of stagnant blood may form in the pocket-shaped atrial appendage and lead to thrombus formation.

Fresh platelets are released from the bone marrow to replace platelets that are used up. Thus, a batch of young platelets is released into the blood after every operation, every childbirth and every injury, to replace the platelets that have been used up. Fresh young platelets tend to stick much more readily than older platelets. It is these sticky young platelets that make the blood particularly liable to form thrombi in the days following operation or childbirth.

In the veins, the common sites for thrombus formation are the deep veins of the pelvis and legs, particularly after abdominal or pelvic operations or childbirth, when the blood flow in these vessels may have been interrupted.

In the arteries, thrombosis occurs mainly where atherosclerosis occurs, that is in the aorta and the major arteries. Thrombosis may also occur in the left ventricle if the lining of the left ventricle is damaged by an infarct.

After a thrombus forms, it may recanalise, or undergo fibrosis, or break away to form an embolus. It may be recanalised either by dissolving away, or by shrinkage of the thrombus. In either case, the lining cells grow in to form a smooth wall to the reformed channel.

If a new passage fails to open up, the thrombus is invaded by granulation tissue. Sometimes the capillaries in the granulation tissue may widen to form new channels through the blockage, but often fibrous tissue predominates and forms a scar, a tough and permanent blockage.

The other possible development is embolus formation.

Embolism

It is from the deep veins of the leg, or pelvis, that thrombi, or parts of thrombi may become detached to form emboli. The blood flow then carries them up the veins to the right side of the heart, and thence into the pulmonary artery (Figure 4-5).

A big embolus can go no further, as the pulmonary artery divides into smaller branches. A big embolus causes a sudden blockage of the pulmonary artery. It is called *Massive Pulmonary Embolism* and death follows within moments, usually with shock.

Smaller pulmonary emboli can pass into the finer branches of the pulmonary arterial tree before jamming and blocking the vessel. This causes a *pulmonary infarct*, with death of the portion of lung tissue affected. The patient suffers a sudden stabbing pain in the side of the chest, and shows a spike of temperature and may cough up a little blood. Whether he survives or not depends on the size of the segment of lung affected, and on whether or not there is only one embolus.

Pulmonary emboli have their origins in the venous system. Systemic emboli

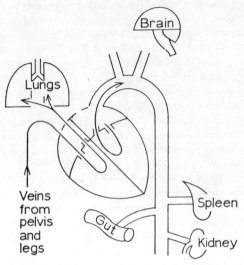

FIG. 4-5 Emboli from the veins go to the lungs. Emboli from the left side of the heart or the arteries may go to any other organ in the body

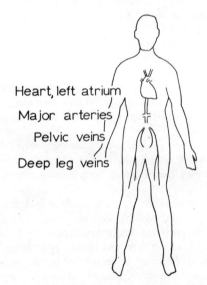

FIG. 4-6 The common sites of thrombus formation which may give rise to emboli

originate in the arteries, or often in the heart itself, especially the left atrial appendage (Figure 4-6). An embolus originating in the left side of the heart is carried in the arterial bloodstream to almost any part of the body, such as the brain, kidneys or spleen.

Other forms of emboli include:

(1) *Septic emboli* which consist of thrombus plus bacteria. They may be detached from the surface of an infected heart valve in bacterial endocarditis and be carried in the arterial blood flow to form an abscess or a mycotic aneurysm at the site where they lodge.

(2) *Air emboli* occur occasionally, due to air bubbles entering the circulation during transfusions or operations, or sometimes due to air bubbles forming in the blood in deep-sea divers who surface too rapidly (Caisson disease or Divers' Bends). The bubbles may act as emboli.

(3) *Fat emboli* occur sometimes following fractures of bones, especially the ribs and the femur. In these cases, many small emboli are formed from fatty bone marrow entering the bloodstream.

(4) *Tumour emboli*, when fragments of a tumour break off into the bloodstream. They are not common, although individual tumour cells are very commonly found in the blood in cancer cases.

(5) Amniotic fluid sometimes enters the mother's blood via the uterine veins during labour, and this may cause numerous pulmonary emboli.

Ischaemia

The term ischaemia means an inadequate blood supply to some part of the body. It is usually due to partial or complete obstruction of an artery. The principal causes are atherosclerosis, thrombosis and embolism. ·

The gradual narrowing of an artery by atherosclerosis is described in Chapter 7. The change leads to a gradual reduction in the blood supply to the part of the body supplied by the artery. It is usually the function of the part that is affected first. For instance, if the coronary arteries that supply the heart muscle are narrowed, the amount of work that the muscle can do becomes limited. It can usually maintain a blood flow that is adequate when the patient is at rest, but it may be incapable of providing an adequate blood flow for any sustained effort, and climbing up flights of stairs becomes impossible.

Later, there may be visible changes in the part supplied; in other words, the form of the part is altered as well as its function. The changes due to ischaemia are seen as scattered areas of necrosis. In the heart muscle, these small areas of cell death are replaced by small fibrous scars, and the change is called diffuse myocardial fibrosis.

Thrombosis and embolism are the other two principal causes of ischaemia. Their effects are different from those of atherosclerosis as they both form complete or nearly complete blockages and also they both occur rapidly. In embolism, the affected artery may be open one moment and completely blocked a moment later. In thrombosis, it may take some hours from the initial platelet plug formation until more platelets, fibrin and cells accumulate to block the artery, but this nevertheless results in a fairly rapid blockage.

In either case, the affected area is more or less suddenly deprived of a blood supply. The result is an infarct. An infarct consists of dead cells. Typically the area has the shape of a wedge or pyramid, with the blockage at the point of the wedge (Figure 4-7).

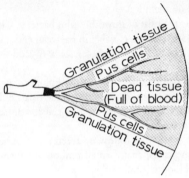

FIG. 4-7   An infarct

The cells affected include the cells in the walls of the small blood vessels, which die and allow the blood cells to escape into the dead tissue. More blood cells may flow into the infarcted area from nearby blood vessels, and this process continues until the area is stuffed with blood cells, and the infarct consists of dead tissue cells and large numbers of blood cells.

Over the following few days, pus cells accumulate at the edge of the infarct and begin to move into the area to digest the dead cells. Also at the edge, in the surrounding living tissue, an inflammatory reaction occurs, and granulation tissue consisting of many small blood vessels and fibre cells develops. By the end of a week or so, provided the patient survives long enough for these changes to occur, the infarct has a soft yellow centre consisting of decomposing tissue and blood cells, and a thin red line at the margin which represents the zone of multiplying small blood vessels. Eventually, after several months perhaps, the dead cells are completely dissolved and digested away, and the fibre cells form a fibrous scar which replaces the dead tissue cells and knits the edges of the area together, like the darning in a hole in a sock.

One factor that may modify the development of an infarct, or even prevent such an occurrence altogether, is the presence of a collateral blood supply. In the wall of the stomach for instance, the arteries that supply the stomach form an intertwining network, and a thrombus or embolus in one artery has little effect as there is always another source of blood supply. For this reason, infarcts of the stomach are almost unheard of. Most of the alimentary tract has a similar form of collateral blood supply, and though infarcts do occur, they are not common.

But some vital organs, such as the brain, the heart and the kidneys, have little effective collateral circulation and in these organs, all too commonly, a thrombus may cause extensive infarction.

A collateral circulation may however develop, at least to some extent. Taking the heart again as an example, it is possible that if one artery is blocked, another one nearby may widen and increase its own blood flow, provided that it too is not already diseased. This process takes time, some months at least, and it is by no means always effective, but certainly in some patients who have survived a coronary artery thrombosis, a collateral blood supply may develop.

GANGRENE

Gangrene is the death of tissue due to poor blood supply. It may occur in infarcted or ischaemic tissue. For example, gangrene is not uncommon in the feet and legs of elderly diabetic patients, due to ischaemia resulting from very severe narrowing of the leg arteries. The tissues of the legs may be so feebly supplied with blood that they offer little or no resistance to bacterial invasion, which may start through some small and insignificant break in the skin.

Gangrene may also occur in tissue that is dead or moribund from other causes. For instance, dead muscle and other tissue may result from an injury, such as a war wound or road traffic accident. Bacterial infection in the dead tissue frequently occurs, and this is also described as gangrene.

5 CANCER

INTRODUCTION

NATURE OF A TUMOUR
Benign and Malignant Tumours
Spread of a Tumour
Some Microscopic Features of Tumour

EFFECTS OF TUMOURS, LOCAL AND GENERAL
Names of Tumours
Diagnosis of Cancer

Treatment of Cancer

CAUSES OF CANCER
Radiation
Chemical Carcinogens
Viruses as a Cause of Cancer
Hormones and Cancer
Heredity
Environment

CANCER INCIDENCE
Cancer and Ageing

Chromosome Abnormalities and Cancer

Cancer and Immunological Mechanisms

Field Theory, Multifactorial and Multistage Theories

DISCUSSION OF CAUSES OF CANCER

INTRODUCTION

Normal growth and development require that the cells of the body multiply in a harmonious and co-ordinated manner. A similar co-ordination is required for the repair of damaged tissues, in foetal development and in pregnancy.

In cancer, the cells of one part of the body multiply excessively, to the detriment of their neighbours and eventually of the whole body.

In inflammation, as we have seen, there is also a considerable multiplication of the cells, but this differs from cancer in that when the stimulus is removed, the inflammation subsides.

NATURE OF A TUMOUR

A tumour is a lump, a new growth or neoplasm. It is made up of cells which in appearance and arrangement resemble the cells of the tissue of origin. Thus a tumour of a gland usually contains some poorly-formed and rather peculiar-looking glandular structures, which can be seen down the microscope.

Normal tissues have a slow and steady turnover of cells, just sufficient to replace the cells that are lost through general wear and tear. Tumour cells multiply more often, and this increases the size of the growth. In general, tumour cells have an increased capacity for multiplication, and a decreased capacity for performing the functions of normal cells.

Tumour cells also show other features, such as loss of contact inhibition. When normal cells are grown in test-tubes they will not grow on top of each other, but cancer cells will. Tumour cells often also show abnormalities of their chromosomes, and another feature of tumour cells is that they usually grow well when transplanted into another animal.

Tumours may grow so rapidly that they outstrip their own blood supply, and soft areas of necrotic tumour cells may be seen. If this occurs at a surface, such as in the skin, then ulceration and infection occur. Areas of haemorrhage are also commonly seen in tumours.

Benign and Malignant Tumours

Benign tumours do not spread. They continue to grow at the site of origin. They form a space-occupying lesion and compress the adjacent tissues. Although they are called benign, they may nevertheless kill the patient if they compress a vital structure such as the trachea.

A tumour is said to be malignant if it spreads. Malignant tumours may spread locally, by forming insidious finger-like projections into the adjacent tissues. Or they may spread more distantly if tumour cells become detached from the original growth and are transported to some distant site in the body to form secondary tumour deposits, called *metastases*. Whether by local invasion, or by forming metastases, this capacity for spread denotes a malignant tumour. The presence of numerous tumour deposits in the body may be referred to as carcinomatosis.

TABLE 5-1 Tumours, benign and malignant

	Benign	Malignant
Growth rate	slow, expansive	rapid
Local invasion	none, usually encapsulated	yes
Distant metastases	none	yes
Recurrence after resection	none	yes
Histology	form—e.g. glandular—preserved function—e.g. keratin formation—preserved	form and function changed
Cytology	normal	abnormal—usually big cells with big irregular nuclei with mitotic figures.
Systemic effects	pressure only	often severe

SPREAD OF A TUMOUR

Tumour cells may spread by being carried to distant sites in the bloodstream. It is by this route that carcinomas of the bronchus may metastasise to the brain or to the liver or elsewhere.

Another route of tumour spread is via the lymphatic channels. In this case the tumour deposits are found in the lymph nodes, such as the lymph nodes in the chest or neck from a bronchial carcinoma (Figure 5-1).

Other routes whereby tumour cells may be spread include the urinary tract, where kidney tumour cells may be carried to the bladder and form secondary deposits there, or body spaces such as the peritoneum where a tumour of the bowel for instance may give rise to numerous tumour seedlings all over the abdominal cavity.

SOME MICROSCOPIC FEATURES OF TUMOUR

When examining the microscopic sections from a tumour, the pathologist may look for various features to help him determine whether a tumour is malignant or not. In a malignant tumour, he might expect to see invasion of the nearby tissues by

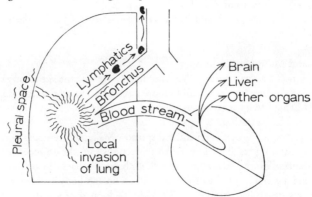

FIG. 5-1 Carcinoma of the bronchus—an example to show the routes by which a malignant tumour may spread

tumour cells, signs of rapid growth and no evidence of a capsule of the compressed surrounding tissues. In general, malignant tumour cells show a greater departure from normal than do the cells of a benign tumour. This applies both to the form and to the function of the cells. Thus, a malignant tumour originating in a gland may show only slight microscopic resemblance to the structure of a normal gland, and there may be no evidence of the production of secretion, which is the function of a normal gland.

EFFECTS OF TUMOURS, LOCAL AND GENERAL

Most pathological processes show both local and general bodily effects, and this is true of tumours.

With tumour, the local effects include obstruction of vital passages such as the gut, and pressure on nearby structures such as blood vessels. This results in the death of the tissues supplied and there may be a severe impairment of function in the affected organ.

TABLE 5-2   Local and systemic effects of cancer

Local	Systemic
Pressure	Anaemia
Obstruction	Cachexia
Haemorrhages	Hormonal
Necrosis	Metastases

The commonest systemic effect of a tumour, whatever its site, is anaemia. This may perhaps be due to the avaricious demand by the tumour cells for protein-building amino acids and other nutriments. *Cachexia* (generalised wasting) may have a similar cause, and so may the decreased level of plasma protein, and the increase in the erythrocyte sedimentation rate.

With some tumours, there occurs an impairment of peripheral nerve function which is not readily accounted for. Other tumours have the capacity to produce substances which act just like normal hormones. For instance, a small number of carcinomas of the bronchus manufacture a cortisone-like substance, the effects of which resemble those of excess cortisone—that is sodium and water retention, trunk oedema and muscle wasting.

NAMES OF TUMOURS

The names of most tumours come from classical Greek, but they do not completely follow any logical plan. We will here only mention a few hints to translators.

Oma means lump—it is used at the ends of the names of most tumours. The first part of the name usually indicates the tissue of origin—e.g. *fibroma* = fibrous tissue lump. The names of malignant tumours usually include the word *carcinoma* if that tumour originates in a surface epithelium (e.g. carcinoma of bronchus) or the word *sarcoma* for tumours arising in connective tissues beneath the surface—e.g. fibro-sarcoma = fibrous tissue malignant lump.

(Other Greek origins are *adeno* = gland, *haem* = blood, *angio* = vessel, *chondro*

= cartilage, *osteo* = bone, *endo* = lining, *myo* = muscle, *leio* = unstriated, *rhabdo* = striated, *terat* = embryo.) Other descriptive words such as follicular or papillary may be used to describe and subdivide the patterns of growth of the many epithelial tumours.

DIAGNOSIS OF CANCER

There can be no diagnosis of cancer until the patient decides to consult his doctor. To encourage this, the seven symptoms listed below have been widely publicised in the U.S.A.

Unusual bleeding or discharge.

A lump or thickening in the breast, or elsewhere.

A sore throat that does not heal.

Change in bowel or bladder habits.

Hoarseness or cough.

Indigestion or difficulty in swallowing.

Change in a wart or a mole.

Clinical examination by the doctor may be sufficient to establish a diagnosis, but further examination is often required, such as:

Instrumental	bronchoscopy, sigmoidoscopy
X-ray	
Cytology	microscopic examination for malignant cells in fluids such as sputum or cervical smears
Surgical biopsy	of a tumour or lymph node suspected of harbouring a secondary tumour deposit
Radioisotope scanning	to identify sites of rapid uptake of radioactive tracer materials

More general investigations may include:

Biochemical tests	for specific or general changes (e.g. acid phosphatase levels in prostatic cancer)
Haematological	for erythrocyte sedimentation rate, anaemia and the like

Treatment of Cancer

Surgical excision is the commonest treatment for cancer and has been for centuries. Provided the diagnosis can be made early enough, it can be highly effective. For instance, two-thirds of all cases of cancer of the cervix are now saved by surgery.

Radiotherapy is less frequently curative, partly because surgery is more commonly used in the early stages. However, in some diseases, such as Hodgkin's disease, a malignant condition of the lymphoid tissue, complete cures are sometimes obtained. Radiotherapy may also be useful as a palliative measure, e.g. to alleviate the pain of secondary tumour deposits in bone.

Many other treatments are used, such as cytotoxic drugs. These are cell poisons.

They include methotrexate, mercaptopurine and cyclophosphamide. They are used in an attempt to poison the rapidly reproducing tumour cells in the body.

Immunotherapy is another method of treatment. Hopeful advances in this field are mentioned later, in the section on Cancer Immunology.

CAUSES OF CANCER

We know of various agents that *can* cause cancer, both in man and in animals, but we do not know what *does* cause cancer in any particular case, nor do we know *how* any of the possible causative factors act.

There are probably many causes of cancer, just as there are many causes of inflammation, and it may be that any one tumour is due not to one cause but to a combination of factors.

Let us consider first some of the factors that are known to be capable of causing tumours.

RADIATION

The changes in cells exposed to ionising radiation are described in Chapter 6. Most of the changes are lethal, and the affected cells die, but an occasional cell may survive with altered characteristics—one of which may be the capacity to form a tumour. Ionising radiation can be used in an attempt to kill off cancer cells, but it may also, on occasions, cause cancer.

Such radiation was the cause of the cancers which developed on the hands of early X-ray workers before they learnt to protect themselves from exposure. Radiation was also responsible for the increased incidence of leukaemia amongst atom-bomb survivors in Japan, and still is responsible for an occasional case of leukaemia amongst patients treated with X-rays for *ankylosing spondylitis*. In such cases there is a latent period of about six years between exposure to the rays and the development of leukaemia.

Another type of radiation, ultraviolet light, is responsible for the high incidence of skin cancers of the face and hands in fair-skinned Australians.

CHEMICAL CARCINOGENS

Over fifty years ago, in 1915, two Japanese gentlemen painted tar on to the skins of rabbits—daubing them twice daily. At first the rabbits' skin went hard, then warts developed which disappeared if the painting was stopped. But if the painting was continued, malignant tumours developed at the site of exposure, and these later spread through the tissues and invaded all parts of the rabbits' bodies.

Since then, this technique has been used many times, to test numerous substances for carcinogenic capacity, and to investigate the effects of the timing and frequency of exposure, and the effects of such other factors as the level of various hormones in the animal's blood.

There is now a lengthy list of chemicals which have been shown by this method to be carcinogenic in animals—such as benzpyrene, dibenzanthracene and 'butter yellow'. These chemicals are sometimes referred to as cancer 'initiators.' A short exposure to one of them produces a latent, but irreversible, potential for tumour development.

Other chemicals such as turpentine or croton oil are sometimes called 'promoters'. By themselves they have an irritant effect, and they do not produce tumours. But prolonged treatment by such irritants has a powerful effect in 'promoting' the appearance of the latent change due to the action of one of the 'initiators'.

A substance called *naphthylamine* is carcinogenic for humans. This substance was used to prevent the rubber in rubber cables from perishing, until it was discovered that some of the workmen developed bladder tumours. Investigations showed that this substance was absorbed, and that it underwent various changes in the body but that it was not until it reached the bladder that it was converted into a carcinogenic substance. After naphthylamine exposure it takes 18 years on average before a bladder tumour develops.

Another substance that is carcinogenic in man is *aflatoxin*. It is produced by a mould that grows on peanuts and groundnuts, and it gives rise to primary liver tumours. It is suspected of having something to do with the high incidence of liver cancers in several countries in Africa.

Other chemical substances strongly suspected of causing cancer in man include some hairdyes and the defoliants used in the Vietnam War. Arsenic which is used in sheep dip and other insecticides can cause skin cancers. Vinyl chloride can give rise to liver tumours in workers in the plastics industry. There is also a considerable suspicion that the high-fat low-residue diets that we eat in the Western world may contribute to our high incidence of bowel and breast cancer.

VIRUSES AS A CAUSE OF CANCER

It would be odd if man were the only animal in whom viruses do not cause tumours. Nobody has yet proved that viruses cause cancer in man, but they certainly do cause cancer in a wide variety of animals.

In 1911, Rous produced tumours in poultry by injecting them with a cell-free juice derived from a fowl tumour. The process took time. After injecting the virus-containing fluid, it took several years before a tumour developed. What happened in this interval is still being investigated.

Since Rous's discovery, numerous other animals have been shown to be affected and numerous other tumour viruses have been found. One interesting virus was originally called *Bittner's milk factor*. Bittner found that the milk of a mother mouse with breast cancer could transmit a factor that caused breast cancer in any female mice that suckled that mother. The subsequent tumours did not appear until the female mice had themselves achieved maturity. The factor was eventually shown to be a virus.

In humans, there has been a good deal of interest recently in *Burkitt's tumour*. It is found in the area around Lake Victoria in Africa. It is a tumour of lymphoid tissue, especially that near the jaws and it occurs mainly in children. It occurs in children of any race, but only in those brought up in an area where the temperature never drops below 13° C and where the annual rainfall is above 20 inches. This distribution strongly suggests that an insect might carry the disease, just as mosquitoes do malaria. Various viruses have been found in extracts from these tumours, and recently a herpes virus called EB virus has been suspected. But the finding of this virus does not prove that it has caused the tumour. It might be purely a coincidence, or the presence of tumour might perhaps in some way encourage virus infection.

There is much speculation as to how viruses cause tumours in animals. Viruses are minute particles that are capable of reproducing, but they can only do this by invading living cells and causing the invaded cells to create new virus material. Viruses thus consist of genetic material, with a thin protective coat, and little more.

When viruses cause diseases such as polio, the invaded cells are eventually killed. In cancer, the cells survive, but the viruses disappear after the initial infection and cannot be found, although the affected cells may develop new antigens which they did not possess before, and which may possibly represent some part of the viruses persisting in the cells.

Somehow or other the viruses affect the genetic material of the cells. Very recently some light has been shed on how the virus inserts its genetic material into the genetic material of the cells. Animal cells use deoxyribonucleic acid (DNA) as the basis of their genetic material. Some tumour viruses also use DNA, but others use a substance called ribonucleic acid (RNA) for theirs. It has recently been shown that the RNA viruses make a RNA-DNA hybrid material as one step in their take-over of the cell's genetic control. It is possible, by sophisticated chemical methods, to detect the RNA-DNA hybrid material in very small quantities. This raises exciting possibilities. One is that by screening human tumour tissue for such traces of viral invasion, it may be possible for the first time to prove that viruses do cause tumours in humans. The second is the even more exciting prospect of being able, by using drugs, to prevent the virus RNA from affecting the cells in this way. A drug that can do this is already known—actinomycin D. Unfortunately, it is very toxic, but perhaps a similar drug can be found that can prevent the viruses from controlling the cells, and then it would really be possible to treat tumours caused by viruses.

HORMONES AND CANCER

Numerous experiments have shown that high levels of hormones, particularly oestrogens, are associated with a high incidence of cancer. Usually the tumour occurs in the normal target organs of the hormones, and the breast is one of the target organs for the oestrogenic hormones. The essential mechanism seems to be a prolonged over-stimulation of the target tissue.

Hormones are generally regarded as promoters of cancer, rather than initiators. Presumably some subtle change must first occur in the cells which, in the presence of persistent hormonal over-stimulation, progresses to tumour formation.

HEREDITY

There is little evidence of an hereditary factor in most human cancers. Six of Napoleon's family are said to have died of carcinoma of the stomach, but this is almost certainly a coincidence and not due to heredity, as carcinoma of the stomach is common, and Napoleon had many relatives.

However, the uncommon tumour of the eye called *Retinoblastoma* does occur more frequently amongst relatives than might be expected from chance, and so do two other uncommon conditions, *multiple polyposis of the colon*, which always develops into malignant cancer unless the whole colon is resected, and the skin condition known as *xeroderma pigmentosum,* which invariably progresses to carcinoma when the skin is exposed to sunlight.

It would therefore appear that for these three rare conditions there is an hereditary tendency, but that for most other human tumours there is little heredity predisposition.

ENVIRONMENT

This is a suitably vague heading under which we may group such topics as cigarette smoking and geographical variations in tumour incidence.

Cigarette smokers alter the internal environment of their bronchi, and all too commonly this is the site of tumour development. There is not the slightest doubt about the fact that people who regularly smoke more than twenty cigarettes a day have a bronchial cancer rate that is over forty times that of non-smokers, and bronchial carcinoma constitutes the number one cancer killer today. There are presumably other factors, as non-smokers occasionally develop bronchial carcinoma, and city dwellers are more liable to it than country folk, but smoking is by far the biggest factor—and one that, in theory at least, could be avoided.

The geographical variations of the incidence of some cancers are very marked—and these are summarised in the sketch map (Figure 5-2).

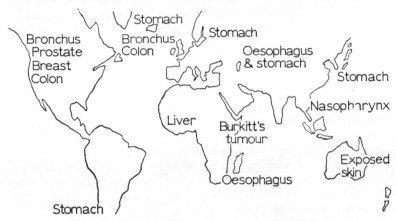

FIG. 5-2 Regions where certain tumours are particularly common

In some cases, factors which might account for these variations are known, such as the strong ultraviolet causing skin tumours in the fair-skinned Australians. But there is complete ignorance about some other tumours. Cancer of the nasopharynx is almost unknown in Europe but is very common among the Chinese of Hong Kong and Singapore. Nitrosamine chemicals in their fermented salt fish have been blamed and also high infection rates by the EB herpes virus.

CANCER INCIDENCE

Cancer is second only to diseases of the heart and blood vessels as a cause of death in the western world, and it accounts for approximately one in five of all deaths. In many parts of the world, however, the old enemies—tuberculosis, malaria,

TABLE 5-3 A summary of the causes of cancer

RADIATION	VIRUSES (in animals)
CHEMICAL CARCINOGENS	HORMONES
e.g. benzpyrene	(Promoting action)
HEREDITY (Rare)	ENVIRONMENT
e.g. multiple polyposis	(Smoking and
of colon	geographic factors)

dysentery and other infections—still take a heavy toll, and in many countries these diseases take first place in the league of killers.

The percentages of all cancer deaths due to common tumours in Britain are shown below, with a few comments in respect of aetiology.

(1)	Trachea, bronchus, lung and pleura	25·0%	Heavy smoking increases the risk forty times
(2)	Stomach	12·2%	Marked geographical variations—Chile, Finland, Japan, all have high rates
(3)	Breast	9·0%	The cow does not get breast cancer, and it has the most overworked mammary gland
(4)	Colon	8·5%	A few cases follow hereditary multiple polyps, others may be related to constipation
(5)	Rectum	5·1%	
(6)	Pancreas	4·3%	
(7)	Prostate	3·6%	
(8)	Bladder	3·3%	Aniline dye workers, and Bilharzia in Egypt
(9)	Ovary	3·0%	
(10)	Leukaemias	2·7%	Atom bomb survivors, various viruses also suspected
(11)	Oesophagus	2·5%	
(12)	Cervix	2·3%	Highest rates where first intercourse early, frequent intercourse, multiple sex partners, low social class. Herpes I and II virus found often. Treatment cures 2 out of 3, so that the incidence rate is 3 times death rate

Cancer and Ageing

The longer you or I live, the greater are the chances that we will develop some types of cancer, namely of oesophagus, stomach, pancreas, rectum, skin and prostate. The incidence of these tumours shows a progressive increase with age.

Other forms of cancer show a different pattern of incidence. They have a peak at a particular age, e.g. cancer of the cervix and breast, and also some leukaemias. For instance carcinoma of the cervix shows a decreased incidence after the age of

50. This is perhaps due to reduction of exposure to some carcinogenic agent, which might be a virus transmitted by sexual intercourse.

Careful study of the incidence of the different forms of cancer at different ages has produced many useful clues about possible cancer causes, just as the study of geographical distribution has done. One interesting result arising from analysis of the figures is the suggestion that the development of cancer from normal tissues requires not one change, but a series of changes. It is, however, much easier to suggest a suspected cause than it is to prove it. The most convincing proof would require the application of a suspected agent to a human being, and demonstrating that it caused cancer. This would be highly unethical, so we must use less direct methods of investigation such as information from animal experiments (which may or may not apply to humans) and information from accidental human exposures, such as the early X-ray workers and their skin carcinomas.

Chromosome Abnormalities and Cancer

Cancer cells often contain an abnormal number of chromosomes. Instead of the usual 46, they may have almost any number—usually more rather than less. These abnormal numbers may be associated with abnormal chromosome patterns when the cells divide. Normal tissues do, very occasionally, show similar abnormal patterns at cell division, but in normal tissues such cells do not survive for long. The cancer cells, however, do survive. It appears therefore that cancer cells have the capacity to survive despite remarkable variations in their chromosome content—and that the capacity for malignant growth implies some degree of independence of chromosomal control. Chromosomal abnormalities therefore are probably not the *cause* of the cancer, but are probably one of the *results* of malignant change.

Cancer and Immunological Mechanisms

The function of the immunological mechanisms is to recognise and react with foreign 'not self' materials.

It is probable that some cancers do not possess any different cell wall proteins from normal cells; they possess no 'foreign' materials for the immunological mechanisms to recognise, and thus no reaction occurs, or could be stimulated to occur.

Other cancers, however, do possess 'foreign' constituents, called 'tumour-associated antigens'. For some reason that is not yet understood, the body does not react sufficiently strongly against these antigens to damage the cancer cells. Mathé in Paris has shown that this immunological deficiency can in some cases be made good. He treats leukaemias by first giving heavy doses of cytotoxic drugs. When, after some months, the number of leukaemic cells in the body has been much reduced, he takes some of the patient's leukaemic cells, irradiates them, and then reinjects them into the patient, together with various adjuvants. By this means he stimulates the body's immunological reaction to its own leukaemic cells, and some at least of his patients have survived for several years already. The crux of this approach appears to be the reduction in the number of tumour cells to a level which the body can be stimulated to react with immunologically.

Field Theory, Multifactorial and Multistage Theories

From animal experiments, and from observations on cancer in humans, it appears that most forms of cancer start not in a single cell but in a group of cells. The appearance is as though a field of cells had all undergone the same change, and certainly in some human cancers it it possible to see cancer-like microscopic changes in the cells near and around the actual tumour.

There is also evidence to suggest that some tumours are due to the effects of several, rather than a single factor. For instance, in some of the skin painting experiments it was found that tumours did not develop unless the animal had at least a certain level of oestrogen hormones in its blood.

These factors may operate together, or one may act before the others in a multistage system to give rise to cancer. In the skin painting experiments again, it was shown that cancers could be produced if an initiator such as methyl cholanthrene were applied several times and then an interval of several months allowed to pass before the promoter (such as turpentine) was applied.

It is possible that some human cancers have a similar multifactorial and multistage origin. We could speculate (and it would be pure speculation) that bronchial carcinoma is initiated by, say, a virus infection in childhood, and that the appearance of a tumour is promoted by subsequent prolonged exposure to tobacco smoke and to a lesser extent the various acids in town chimney smoke.

This kind of complication makes cancer research a very complex subject.

DISCUSSION OF CAUSES OF CANCER

Normal growth and development depends on a number of control mechanisms—control within the cell, mostly by the genes, controls such as contact inhibition between adjacent cells by physical factors, local chemical control in a group of cells by chalones and local metabolite concentrations, and more generalised controls by circulating hormones and nervous stimulation, and during development by various postulated chemical inducing and organising mechanisms. And there is also the immunological control mechanism, by means of cells or circulating chemical antibodies, which recognise and react against any foreign 'not self' material that may appear within the body. The body, therefore, has a complicated system of controls for the development of and maintenance of you and me as individual human beings.

Cancer cells arise from normal controlled cells, but they do not respond to one or more of the control mechanisms. This is the basic abnormality of cancer cells. It appears always to be linked to a change in the genetic make-up of the cell, as tumour cells transmit their neoplastic character to their daughter cells.

Many other changes may sometimes be present in cancer cells, such as reduced generation time, lack of contact inhibition, new antigenic properties (tumour associated antigens), abnormal cell forms, abnormal number or pattern of chromosomes, altered cell function, occasionally including the acquisition of new bizarre functions such as secretion of hormone-like chemicals, and the ability to survive and multiply in foreign surroundings (metastases). All these and other changes may be seen in tumour cells and they determine the character of the tumour. But it is the genetic change associated with unresponsiveness to one or more of the control mechanisms which appears to be common to all tumours, and without which there would be no cancer.

It is possible that small changes occur from time to time in the genetic material of one or two of the millions and millions of cells in the body. Most of such changes probably so alter the function of the cell as to be lethal and not transmitted. It would only be the very occasional change that would confer independence of the control mechanisms we have mentioned. The precise nature of this change is the central mystery of cancer.

6 MISCELLANEOUS DISEASE PROCESSES

AMYLOIDOSIS

CONGENITAL AND HEREDITARY DISORDERS
Congenital Disorders

Hereditary Disorders

Chromosome Examination

Chromosome Abnormalities
Turner's Syndrome
Klinefelter's Syndrome

Genetic Defects—Inborn Errors of Metabolism
Cystic Fibrosis
Haemophilia

HYPOTHERMIA AND FROSTBITE

NUTRITIONAL DISORDERS
Scurvy and Multiple Vitamin Deficiencies
Kwashiorkor
Obesity

THE EFFECTS OF IONISING RADIATION
Radiation Sickness
Scarring
Necrosis
Bone Necrosis

AMYLOIDOSIS

Amyloidosis is a curious and not very common condition in which there is a deposition of white waxy material in the walls of the small blood vessels and in the liver, kidney and spleen and occasionally in the heart. These organs may be packed with amyloid material and partly destroyed by it, and occasionally death occurs from hepatic or renal failure, but this is rare. The material is mainly a glycoprotein.

Nobody knows the cause of amyloidosis, although it does appear to be associated with conditions in which abnormally high levels of antibodies are produced. It is seen, for instance, as a complication of rheumatoid arthritis and in multiple myelomatosis, in both of which conditions large quantities of abnormal antibodies are present in the blood. It may also occur in association with chronic infections such as bronchiectasis or chronic osteomyelitis, though these conditions are less commonly seen now than in pre-antibiotic days.

CONGENITAL AND HEREDITARY DISORDERS

Congenital Disorders

A congenital disorder is something a person is born with, a disease due to influences *in utero*, such as congenital syphilis, which is acquired during foetal development from an infected mother. Other examples are the congenital defects due to the mother's exposure to thalidomide or German measles during pregnancy.

Hereditary Disorders

The hereditary disorders originate from a fertilised ovum which has an abnormal chromosomal or genetic constitution. All the cells in the person that develops from that fertilised ovum are affected by the abnormality.

Normally the fertilised ovum contains 23 pairs of chromosomes, of which 22 single chromosomes and one sex chromosome (an X chromosome) are present in the unfertilised ovum derived from the mother, and 22 single chromosomes plus one sex chromosome (which is either another X chromosome, or is a smaller Y chromosome) are present in the sperm. A fertilised ovum with a Y chromosome develops into an individual with male characteristics, and a fertilised ovum without a Y chromosome (and that is normally an ovum with two X chromosomes) develops into a female (Figure 6-1).

Chromosome Examination

It is possible to see the chromosomes in cells down the microscope, and leucocytes from a blood specimen are usually used for this purpose. It is possible to detect abnormal numbers of chromosomes or misshapen chromosomes. Recently-developed staining techniques using atebrin have made it possible to identify each of the 23 pairs of chromosomes and to give them numbers, and thus to pinpoint which chromosome abnormalities are responsible for particular bodily disorders.

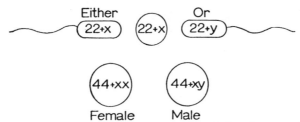

FIG. 6-1 The sex of an individual depends on whether the sperm that fertilises the ovum contains an X or a Y chromosome

Chromosome Abnormalities

Mongols are the commonest living examples of chromosomal abnormalities. One child in six hundred is a Mongol. They are innocent and happy mental defectives, with hyperextensible joints, rather flat heads and slant eyes with prominent epicanthic folds. Instead of the usual two chromosomes numbered 21, Mongols have three (Trisomy 21). The extra chromosome derives from an abnormal ovum and this abnormality is much more likely to occur if the mother is more than 35 years old.

Other fairly common chromosomal abnormalities are those involving the sex chromosomes.

TURNER'S SYNDROME

The cells of these patients show that they only have a single sex chromosome, an X chromosome. They are all females as they have no Y chromosome, but they have no effective ovaries and are infertile. As with most chromosomal abnormalities, they show a multiplicity of abnormalities, including short stature, often mental subnormality, and a curious webbing of the neck.

It may be of interest to note that at least a third of all spontaneous abortions show chromosomal abnormalities, and that a quarter of these are Turner's syndrome (XO). Thus, to a certain extent nature operates a quality control system by aborting some pregnancies with chromosomal abnormalities.

KLINEFELTER'S SYNDROME

These people are males with an XXY sex chromosome pattern, i.e. they are male because they have a Y chromosome, and abnormal because of the extra X chromosome. These men have small testes, no sperms and they have rather long arms and legs.

Genetic Defects—Inborn Errors of Metabolism

The majority of hereditary stigmas occur when the chromosome pattern is entirely normal, but where one gene on one of the chromosomes is abnormal. When a single gene is defective, it fails to order the production of the enzyme needed for a single biochemical process, and such single gene defects are called inborn errors of metabolism (Figure 6-2).

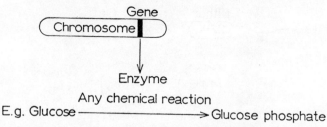

FIG. 6-2   Each biochemical reaction within a cell is controlled by one of the
thousand or more genes on one of the chromosomes

CYSTIC FIBROSIS

Cystic fibrosis, which causes abnormal secretion by various glands (see Chapter 13),
is the most common inborn error of metabolism, and is found in about one out of
every thousand children. Probably about one person in fifty unwittingly carries one
such defective gene, but the disease of cystic fibrosis only occurs if the genes derived
from both the parents are defective.

HAEMOPHILIA

Haemophilia (see Chapter 4) is due to a defect of the gene that codes for the production of anti-haemophilic globulin. This gene is located on the X sex chromosome. The disease haemophilia only occurs if there is no other X chromosome with
a normal gene on it. Males only have one X chromosome, which they inherit from
their mothers. If the single X chromosome carries a defective gene, then they have
haemophilia. The condition is sex-linked in that it can only affect males, who
acquire the defective genes from their unaffected mothers.

OTHER ERRORS

Other similar inborn errors of metabolism include **phenylketonuria,** in which
severe mental retardation occurs due to the accumulation of toxic levels of phenyl-
alanine, and achondroplasia, a variety of dwarfism which may be seen in most
circuses. It is just possible that **schizophrenia** may eventually turn out to be another
inborn error of metabolism, involving the substance 6-hydroxydopamine.

Other defects such as spina bifida, hare lip and diabetes mellitus are probably
also due to defective genes. These disorders are considered to be multifactorial,
in that more than one abnormal gene is involved.

HYPOTHERMIA AND FROSTBITE

In hypothermia, the body temperature drops. When this happens, all the chemical
processes in the body become slower, and even the mental processes are sluggish.
Somewhere between 29° and 32° C, small thrombi begin to form in many of the
small blood vessels throughout the body. Many organs are damaged in the process
and unless the patient is speedily rescued, death from cardiac arrest is likely to
follow, due to a combination of myocardial damage and peripheral circulatory
collapse.

This situation is seen in old people and occasionally in babies, and is due to a combination of very cold winter weather, lack of fuel to keep the house warm overnight, and inability to take any exercise to generate body heat.

In frostbite, the central body temperature is not changed, but the circulation may be inadequate to maintain the temperature of exposed parts such as the cheeks and extremities. This happens in Britain in wintry weather, when people get their gloves or feet wet while out in the mountains. Any wind blowing increases the rate of cooling by evaporation. (Incidentally, a large thin plastic bag which can be slipped on the limb, under the wet clothing, is very effective in reducing the heat loss in such circumstances.) If the exposed part is allowed to cool, numerous small thrombi form in the blood vessels. The skin and other tissues do not immediately die, as they are refrigerated, but they may do so when the temperature is restored to normal, as the thrombi persist and the tissue is ischaemic and necrotic and may very easily become infected (gangrene).

NUTRITIONAL DISORDERS

Nutritional disorders are usually due to a deficient intake of food in relation to the body's needs. It may be noted that these needs are increased during growth and pregnancy. Nutritional disorders may also occur as a result of defects of digestion or absorption, such as deficiency of Vitamin B_{12} due to absence of intrinsic factor, or deficiency of protein and fat-soluble vitamins in malabsorption (Chapter 11).

The dietary deficiencies seen in Britain include iron-deficiency anaemia (Chapter 9), vitamin D deficiency in rickets and osteomalacia (Chapter 17), iodine deficiency with simple colloid goitre (Chapter 16) and scurvy and multiple vitamin deficiencies.

SCURVY AND MULTIPLE VITAMIN DEFICIENCIES

Scurvy is basically a deficiency of ascorbic acid (vitamin C), a vitamin that is present in most fresh fruits, especially oranges, lemons, tomatoes and black currants. Cooking destroys vitamin C.

The people most liable to develop scurvy are those who eat no fruit, such as old people, especially men living alone, or tramps. Apart from poverty, one reason why they eat no fruit is that they may have no teeth. These patients are usually severely enfeebled by anaemia, and they may show numerous tiny haemorrhages in the skin, often first appearing on the thighs. The most characteristic change is in the gums which are markedly swollen and liable to bleed.

In Britain, the people liable to develop scurvy are also liable to other nutritional deficiencies. It is rare for a single deficiency to be present. Patients with multiple vitamin deficiencies may have sores around the mouth, curious neurological defects, osteomalacia and even nutritional oedema due to protein deficiency.

KWASHIORKOR

Kwashiorkor is not seen in Britain, except in television news programmes, but it is unfortunately all too common elsewhere. It affects children, particularly between 1 and 5 years old, and it is principally due to severe and prolonged deficiency of protein. In tropical countries, particularly in war-scarred areas, children may exist on a diet of nothing but starchy gruel. Any infection, such as hookworm infestation, malaria or measles may precipitate kwashiorkor, due to the increase in protein requirements.

These children do not grow, and they show marked muscle wasting which is most obvious in the face and arms, as the wasting of the trunk and legs is often obscured by severe oedema. A curious change, from which apparently the disease gets its name, is that the hair may change colour from black to grey or even orange.

OBESITY

The commonest nutritional disorder in western countries is obesity, in which there is an excessive deposition of fat in the body, mostly in the subcutaneous tissues. It can be defined by weight measurements, as 10 per cent or more over the standard weights for persons of the same age, sex and stature, or by measurements with skin callipers of the thickness of the subcutaneous fat.

Excess body fat serves no useful purpose. It acts as a dead weight. A person who is 1 stone (7 kg) overweight has to move 1 stone of extra weight with every movement, whether it be turning over in bed or climbing a flight of stairs. The effect can be likened to a normal person who chooses to carry fourteen 1-lb bags of sugar around in his pockets everywhere he goes. No offence is intended to the Women's Lib. movement in pointing out that women normally have more subcutaneous fat than men, and that there are many more obese women than men. Scotland certainly has its share of small women who may weigh 8 stones (56 kg) at the time of marriage, but who weigh 16 stones (112 kg) twenty years later.

The cause of obesity is too much food, or too little exercise, or both together. An hormonal imbalance, such as Cushing's syndrome, is sometimes suspected but this diagnosis is only very rarely confirmed.

We tend to eat more food than we require for our energy needs, especially carbohydrates such as bread, potatoes, cereals, cakes, biscuits, sugar, beer and spirits. The problem is, why do we eat so much? Psychological factors probably come into it. Two-thirds of all cases of obesity are middle-aged women, and it may be that boredom, or the real or supposed lack of other sources of satisfaction, drive them to the cakes and pastries. Many women eat too much, and they get fatter for a while until the increased energy required to shift their extra weight around catches up with the food intake, after which time they maintain a fairly constant but excessive body weight. It may be also that our inborn desire for food has not adjusted to modern life. Only a few generations ago, walking was the main method of transport, and walking uses up 300 calories per hour, and even more recently, efficient methods of heating have largely deprived us of the task of keeping ourselves warm.

Obesity reduces the expectancy of life. Fat men, between the ages of 20 and 64, have a death rate that is one and a half times that of thin men. The higher death rate is due to an increased incidence of atherosclerosis, myocardial infarction, hypertension and hypertensive kidney disease. Apart from the increased risk of death, obesity brings many obstacles to the proper enjoyment of life, including increased incidences of angina pectoris, cardiac failure, diabetes mellitus, gallstones, varicose veins, hiatus hernia, degenerative joint disease (osteoarthrosis) and poor respiration which predisposes to chronic bronchitis.

There are other important causes of weight increase, notably oedema and pregnancy.

THE EFFECTS OF IONISING RADIATION

Ionising radiation comes from the sun, from radioactive materials such as isotopes, from atomic bombs and from X-ray machines, and we are all exposed to a low degree all the time from naturally occurring radioactive materials in the soil. Ionising radiation alters the make-up of any atom it hits by moving or removing one of the electrons. An ionised atom instantaneously acquires different chemical affinities from a normal atom, and rapid and powerful changes therefore occur in any cell exposed to ionising radiation. Most of such changes are lethal to the cell and the affected cell dies, but an occasional cell may survive with altered characteristics, one of which may be the capacity to form a tumour.

Thus ionising radiation may be used therapeutically in an attempt to kill off cancer cells, but it may also occasionally cause cancer.

In general, rapidly multiplying cells are more susceptible to ionising radiation than less active cells. Rapidly multiplying tumour cells can thus be mostly killed, while the adjacent normal cells may be relatively little affected. However, we all have other rapidly multiplying cells in our bodies, particularly the cells lining the intestines and the blood-forming cells in the bone marrow. These are particularly liable to be affected by ionising radiation, and as a precaution, radiotherapy staff members have regular blood checks of their blood platelet and white cell counts.

Radiotherapy is sometimes effective in arresting a rapidly growing tumour, although it is seldom possible to destroy all the tumour cells completely. In many cases, radiotherapy can give considerable relief from the pain caused by tumour secondaries. In other cases, such as osteosarcoma, the arrest produced by radiotherapy may allow a surgical removal to be performed, and in some cases of Hodgkin's disease and seminoma of the testis, radiotherapy has produced a complete and lasting cure.

The methods used in radiotherapy are such that the risk of a tumour arising as a result of treatment is now very small, but other complications are, however, sometimes seen.

RADIATION SICKNESS
Radiation sickness is not common now. It is a form of nausea and malaise, probably due to excessive tissue destruction releasing large amounts of protein-split products into the circulation all at once.

SCARRING
The connective tissue cells and the blood vessels in an area exposed to radiation undergo changes leading to extensive fibrosis, and in the intestines, for instance, such scars can give rise to troublesome obstructions.

NECROSIS

The skin and other tissues in the path of the radiation may suffer, and in some cases the skin cells die and fall away. Subsequent healing or skin grafting may be very difficult, and take years to achieve because of the fibrosis and vascular changes in the surrounding tissues.

BONE NECROSIS

Bones show up well on X-rays because they absorb more radiation than the other tissues; for the same reason bones are more liable to be damaged by radiation than other tissues. Usually the damage takes the form of bone necrosis, but very occasionally a bone tumour may originate at the radiation site.

7 DISEASES OF THE BLOOD VESSELS AND HYPERTENSION

DISEASES OF THE LARGE ARTERIES
Atherosclerosis

Main Effects of Atherosclerosis
Thrombosis
Ischaemia
Aneurysm Formation
Dissecting Aneurysm

Causes of Atherosclerosis
Level of Cholesterol and Neutral Fat in the Blood
Fatty Streaking
Fibrin Deposition

Summary of the Causes of Atherosclerosis

Syphilitic Aortitis

DISEASES OF THE MEDIUM-SIZED ARTERIES
Monckberg's Sclerosis
Buerger's Disease
Giant Cell Arteritis

DISEASES OF THE SMALL ARTERIES
Polyarteritis Nodosa
Raynaud's Phenomenon
Raynaud's Disease
Thrombotic Microangiopathy

ANEURYSMS

TUMOURS OF BLOOD VESSELS
Capillary Angioma
Glomangioma
Haemangioma

DISEASES OF THE VEINS
Varicose Veins
Varicose Ulcers
Thrombophlebitis

Haemorrhoids (Piles)
Varicocele

Deep Leg-vein Thrombosis

HYPERTENSION

DISEASES OF THE LARGE ARTERIES
Atherosclerosis
Atherosclerosis is by far the most important disease of the arteries, as about a quarter of all the deaths in the western world are due to its effects. We will consider the nature of atherosclerosis first, and its main effects, before going on to consider its possible causes.

A normal artery has a glistening smooth inner lining and a strong flexible wall. In atherosclerosis, the lining is damaged and the wall may also be damaged.

Atherosclerosis is often called 'hardening of the arteries' but there is more to it than that. It affects the aorta and its main branches, and consists of hard, rough, yellow patches which develop in the lining of these vessels. The patches are called plaques, and *atheroma* is the name given to the combination of substances which make up the plaques. These are cholesterol, neutral fats and fibrin.

Cholesterol and neutral fats are fatty substances which normally circulate in the blood. Fibrin circulates dissolved in the blood as fibrinogen. Normally it is only turned into fibrin when coagulation of the blood is necessary to prevent bleeding, but in atherosclerosis fibrin is formed where it serves no useful purpose.

Later, two other constituents may be added, fibrous scar tissue made by fibro-blast cells, and calcium. Fibrous scar tissue gradually replaces some of the deposits of fibrin, and stony hard calcium may also be deposited, so that, at post-mortem examination, the arteries crackle and shatter like egg-shells. In some places the hard deposits in the lining of the artery may prevent the proper nutrition from reaching parts of the artery wall. The cells in these areas of the artery walls die and leave soft patches which may ulcerate.

Atherosclerosis, then, is a patchy degeneration of the lining of the large arteries, in which rough hard plaques of atheroma are formed, and may be associated with soft or ulcerated areas. Cholesterol, neutral fats and fibrin are the main constituents of atheroma, to which fibrous tissue and calcium deposits may later be added.

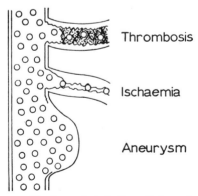

FIG. 7-1 The three principal effects of atherosclerosis

Main Effects of Atherosclerosis

THROMBOSIS

The general features of arterial thrombosis have been previously described (Chapter 4). Thrombus formation is common and often fatal. A plaque of atheroma in the normally smooth lining of an artery disturbs the steady flow of blood; this, and the roughness of the surface of the plaque, often cause the blood to clot. A thrombus which forms on a plaque in an important vessel may completely block the passage of blood and lead to an infarct. The coronary arteries, the internal carotid and the cerebral arteries are the most commonly affected, and thrombus formation in these vessels often cause infarcts in the heart or brain. Such a heart attack or stroke is always serious and often fatal.

ISCHAEMIA

The hard plaques of atheroma may make the arteries narrow and reduce the volume of blood that can flow in them. This condition of shortage of blood supply is called ischaemia. It can affect any part of the body but is most commonly noticed in two places: the heart and the legs. In the heart, the condition is known as *Angina pectoris*. In this condition the coronary arteries are the ones narrowed by atherosclerosis. The amount of blood that reaches the heart muscle is enough for the patient when he is sitting down, or asleep in bed, but the blood supply is not enough for the heart when a load is placed on it, such as in exercise. Thus when the patient climbs up stairs or runs for a bus, particularly in cold weather, he is seized by a gripping pain in the chest and is forced to stop and wait until the supply of blood to the heart can catch up with the demand. All his activities are therefore limited by the state of his coronary arteries.

The situation is similar in the legs, and here it is given the name of *Intermittent claudication*. The leg muscles need a good blood supply for their normal work. An 8-stone (50 kg) person weighs a hundredweight, the same as a sack of coal. For each step that person takes, he must lift a hundredweight and put it down again in another place, and if he happens to be climbing a hill at the time the task is even harder. Not surprisingly, patients in whom the arteries to the legs are clogged by atherosclerosis suffer cramp-like pain in the legs when walking, particularly when walking uphill. The pain may be severe, and such patients learn to stop and pretend to look into shop windows until the pain passes off, and they can resume their journey.

ANEURYSM FORMATION

This is the third and last of the serious conditions which may develop as a result of atherosclerosis. If the inner part of the wall of an artery is weakened by atherosclerosis, it may give way. The pressure of the blood then pushes against the outer wall, which stretches and is slowly pushed out to form a balloon-like bag, an aneurysm. The common sites for this to happen are the abdominal part of the aorta and the cerebral arteries. It is no secret that the late Duke of Windsor successfully underwent an operation in which an abdominal aortic aneurysm was removed, and a flexible teflon tube was put in, to replace the damaged part of the aorta.

Aneurysms are fairly common as a result of atherosclerosis but not as common as thromboses or ischaemic effects.

You might imagine that an aneurysm exposed to the persistent pounding of the pressure waves of the pulse would get bigger and bigger until eventually it burst. This can and does happen, especially in the cerebral arteries where it results in a subarachnoid haemorrhage. The reason why most aneurysms do not rupture is that a thrombus often forms, due to clotting of the blood in the aneurysm. The thrombus is not very strong, but is strong enough to prevent rupture of some aneurysms.

DISSECTING ANEURYSM

Thick deposits of atheroma in the lining of the aorta may prevent the proper nutrition from reaching the cells of the middle layer of the wall of the aorta and many of the cells in this layer may die. This leaves the diseased inner layer of the wall very feebly connected to the outer layer, a tube within a tube. If the inner wall has a weak patch in it which breaks down, blood can escape through the hole and push its way between the inner and outer tubes, giving rise to the curious form of aneurysm called a dissecting aneurysm.

The escaped blood may force its way for quite a distance between the layers of the wall of the aorta, and cause a sometimes bewildering variety of signs and symptoms. The tearing apart of the two layers of the vessel wall causes severe pain in the chest or abdomen, and the patient may in fact describe it as a tearing sensation. The presence of blood or thrombus in the wall of the aorta may distort the other arteries where they branch off, and thus the pulse in an arm or a leg may be reduced. Death commonly occurs due to rupture of the outer layer of the wall of the aorta, with massive haemorrhage into the chest or abdominal cavities.

Everybody develops atherosclerosis as they grow older, and the effects described above are frequently seen. But it should be pointed out that many people have severe atherosclerosis but show none of the three serious effects mentioned.

Causes of Atherosclerosis

There is no single cause of atherosclerosis. Numerous factors are known to play a part in causing it, and a large amount of research work has been done on these factors, but it is difficult to determine exactly what part each of the various factors plays, or how they fit into the complex process known as atherosclerosis.

LEVEL OF CHOLESTEROL AND NEUTRAL FAT IN THE BLOOD

It is known that people with high levels of cholesterol and neutral fat in their blood tend to get more severe atherosclerosis, and it is also known that, at least in some groups of people, a high fat diet raises the blood levels of these substances. A high sugar diet may do the same. The level of cholesterol in the blood is also higher than normal in two common conditions, *Diabetes mellitus* and *Myxoedema*. Patients with either of these conditions suffer more severe atherosclerosis than normal people.

FATTY STREAKING

No one knows why some of the cholesterol and neutral fat from the blood should be deposited in the linings of the arteries, but nevertheless it is, and the higher the levels in the blood, the more cholesterol and neutral fat is dumped in the lining of the arteries. This tendency is very much increased in patients with high blood pressures. The deposits show as yellow fatty streaks in the linings of the arteries. Nearly everyone over the age of 15 has some of these fatty streaks.

FIBRIN DEPOSITION

Fibrin, the main chemical substance concerned in the coagulation of the blood, is deposited as a crust on some of the fatty streaks. Factors which favour the accumulation of fibrin include fatty meals, smoking and lack of exercise, all of which probably act not so much by encouraging fibrin deposition as by slowing down fibrinolysis, which is the chemical process by which fibrin is removed. Much of the fibrin deposited is eventually replaced by tough fibrous tissue.

Summary of the Causes of Atherosclerosis

The factors that have already been mentioned include age, diet (especially high fat diets), myxoedema, diabetes, high blood pressure, lack of exercise and tobacco smoking. A possible way in which these factors may be related is shown in the diagram (Figure 7-2).

Other factors that are involved in atherosclerosis production are:

Sex—Being female is a great advantage as, for some unknown reason, women seldom develop much atherosclerosis until after the menopause. After the age of 45

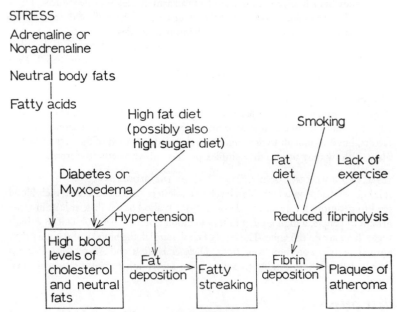

FIG. 7-2 A scheme showing how various factors may combine in the development of atherosclerosis

or so, the advantage is lost, and by the age of 70 there is no difference between the sexes.

Stress—Emotional stress is probably a significant factor in causing atherosclerosis. Perhaps the effect of stress involves the hormones adrenaline and noradrenaline. It is known that we secrete more of these hormones into the blood during stressful activities such as driving in the rush-hour traffic. These two hormones mobilise free fatty acids from the neutral fat stores under the skin. The primitive hunting man would have promptly utilised the free fatty acids to provide energy to chase an animal or run away from it. Civilised man cannot dispose of free fatty acids so easily. The only muscular activity he has is to toot his car horn in exasperation, while the free fatty acids in his blood are slowly converted back into neutral fat, and, perhaps, deposited in the walls of his arteries.

The most important features of atherosclerosis are its effects, thrombosis, ischaemia and to lesser extent aneurysm formation. These effects kill so many people that it is not surprising that a good deal of effort has been put into trying to determine why cholesterol, neutral fats and fibrin should be deposited in the walls of the arteries. As we have seen, numerous factors are concerned, and it is only by further research that we can hope to learn how to prevent this major disease.

Syphilitic Aortitis
Syphilis can nearly always be cured in its early stages by pencillin, and so syphilitic aortitis, which occurs in one of the later stages of the disease is now only rarely seen. It mainly affects the arch of the aorta, where numerous small pearly thickenings form in the lining. This has somewhat flippantly been called 'the pearly arch of Venus'. The pearly thickenings may grow and fuse together, and some of the underlying muscle in the wall of the aorta may become soft and die. The weakened part of the wall of the aorta may, as in atherosclerosis, give way and balloon out to form an aneurysm. Thus syphilis can be a cause of aortic aneurysm, but it is uncommon.

DISEASES OF THE MEDIUM-SIZED ARTERIES
The medium-sized arteries do not often become diseased. Three conditions are mentioned briefly here. You may one day see a case, but they are all rare, and no cause is known for any of them.

MONCKBERG'S SCLEROSIS
Monckberg's sclerosis affects arteries such as the radial artery at the wrist, at the place where it is customary to feel the pulse. Heavy deposits of chalky material are laid down in the walls of these arteries, which look like and feel like the stems of clay pipes.

BUERGER'S DISEASE
Buerger's disease affects men, mainly in the arteries of the legs. The linings of the medium-sized arteries become very much thickened by granulation tissue, which

partially or completely blocks the arteries, and may lead to gangrene in the toes or legs. Cigarette smoking certainly makes it worse, but the cause is unknown.

GIANT CELL ARTERITIS

The temporal artery (where you can feel the pulse against the bone just in front of the ear) is the usual site of Giant Cell Arteritis and the disease is sometimes referred to as Temporal Arteritis. The artery becomes blocked by granulation tissue in which there are usually many giant cells. The patients are nearly always over 60, and they develop a throbbing pain in the temples, which often subsides after six months or so. In a few cases however, the vessels to the retina of the eye are affected and they may go blind, and in a very small number of cases the arteries supplying the brain are also affected, and these patients may die of cerebral infarction.

DISEASES OF THE SMALL ARTERIES

The small arteries are often involved in areas of inflammation (Chapter 2). They may also be involved in several diseases which affect the whole of the body such as diabetes, syphilis and systemic lupus erythematosus (described elsewhere). Diseases of the small arteries themselves are uncommon, but they are important enough to deserve mention.

POLYARTERITIS NODOSA

This disease gets its name from the little nodes or lumps that develop along the courses of many of the small and some of the medium-sized arteries. Each node is a small aneurysm that forms where a small part of the wall is weakened in a patch of intense inflammation. No one knows what causes these small patches of inflammation. Thrombus formation is liable to occur on each of these patches, with blockage of the artery and development of a small infarct, and haemorrhage may also occur as some of the aneurysms rupture into the surrounding tissues. There may be five hundred or more of the small aneurysms, each about the size of a pinhead, scattered throughout the body, and the clinical findings may be very odd. They may include changes in the brain, skin and lungs, as well as in the kidneys. The kidneys are most commonly affected, with blood and protein in the urine. A biopsy of one of the lesions is usually the best method of diagnosis. Death may occur, following damage to any of the bodily systems involved.

RAYNAUD'S PHENOMENON

This is not really a disease at all; it is an exaggeration of the narrowing of the small arteries which occurs normally when they are exposed to cold. In cold weather, the arteries contract so much that the fingers, toes, ears and nose may go white and 'dead', but they eventually recover after warming and there is no residual damage.

RAYNAUD'S DISEASE

This is very similar, but in these cases there is residual damage. The damage is caused by thrombus formation in the contracted vessels. It starts as blistering of the skin and may progress to ulceration of the fingertips.

THROMBOTIC MICROANGIOPATHY—THROMBOTIC THROMBOCYTOPENIC PURPURA

The two long-winded names of this uncommon condition indicate some of its features. The smallest arteries and the arterioles become plugged by tiny thrombi formed mainly of fibrin and platelets. Small infarcts are produced in many areas, and there may be many small haemorrhages, especially in the brain. The cause is unknown. The effects include fever, deficiency of platelets, bizarre neurological changes and often death.

ANEURYSMS

One of the commonest kinds of aneurysm is a *berry aneurysm*, so called because it looks like a berry growing on the twigs of the cerebral arterial tree. Berry aneurysms form at sites where there is some slight congenital weakness in the wall of the cerebral arteries. A plaque of atherosclerosis may similarly weaken the wall. The pressure of the blood, particularly if the pressure is higher than normal, then balloons out the aneurysm. Berry aneurysms frequently rupture, with haemorrhage either into the brain or into the subarachnoid space.

Bacteria carried in an infected embolus may attack the wall of an artery from within, and give rise to another kind of aneurysm called a *mycotic aneurysm*. The commonest source for such infected emboli is an infected heart valve in bacterial endocarditis.

The aneurysms that may occur in atherosclerosis, syphilitic aortitis and poly-arteritis nodosa have been described earlier.

TUMOURS OF BLOOD VESSELS
Capillary Angioma

These lesions consist of collections of small vessels full of blood in the skin. They usually lie flat in the skin and look as though the patient has spilled some black-currant juice on his face or elsewhere. Sometimes they project above the skin and look rather like small strawberries. Both kinds are entirely benign, although the patient may be self-concious about these birthmarks.

GLOMANGIOMA

This is a small knot of blood vessels found in the fingers, often under the finger nail. It is benign but may be very painful.

HAEMANGIOMA

These tumours of blood vessels are rare. They may occur in the liver, the cere-bellum or elsewhere. They may bleed or press on some important structure.

DISEASES OF THE VEINS
Varicose Veins

The pressure of the blood coming from the capillaries into the veins is small, and so there is only a small pressure to push the blood along. The rate of blood flow is therefore normally small in the veins, and this is especially true of the blood in the leg veins which, when we stand up, has a long uphill journey to return to the heart. When we walk about, the muscles of our legs alternately expand and contract, and each expansion squeezes the nearby veins. Because the veins have flap-like one-way valves, this squeezing helps to move the blood towards the heart. If, however, we stand still for a long time, this pumping action is lost, and the veins in the legs become distended with blood. The walls of the veins may then be stretched by the pressure, giving rise to an ache, and if the process is often repeated, varicose veins may be the result.

Varicose veins are blue snakey bulges beneath the skin. Good examples can be seen in most bus queues. They occur most commonly in the superficial veins of the legs in people such as nurses and bartenders who may spend many hours each day standing more or less still. Varicose veins look ugly and they frequently ache, but seldom give rise to serious trouble, although an injury to such a vein may cause severe bleeding.

VARICOSE ULCERS (GRAVITATIONAL ULCERS)
In some people, varicose veins may seriously interfere with the return of blood from the skin of the legs. The skin is taut and shiny and has a blue-brown colour. Any slight injury is sufficient to break the skin, and because of the poor blood flow, healing is very slow and bacterial infection and ulceration are common.

THROMBOPHLEBITIS
The wall of a vein in the vicinity of a varicose ulcer, or after a knock, may become inflamed and thrombus formation is common in the inflamed area. Thrombosed superficial veins never, or almost never, give rise to the release of emboli.

HAEMORRHOIDS (PILES)
Haemorrhoids are varicose veins at the anus. These veins may become distended by straining to empty the bowel, or by damage to the delicate epithelium caused by the passage of stony hard faecal material. Thrombosis of the distended veins may be followed by fibrosis and healing, or the haemorrhoids may persist and require surgical removal. They may also bleed.

VARICOCELE
Varicose veins in the spermatic cord are called varicoceles. Usually no underlying cause is found for this condition.

Deep Leg-vein Thrombosis
The deep veins of the legs include the femoral veins and the veins deep in the muscles. These veins are separate from the superficial veins, and thrombosis of these deep veins is caused by different factors from thrombosis of the superficial veins. The factors include bed rest, in which the venous blood flow is reduced generally, pregnancy, childbirth, and operations in the abdomen or pelvis in which slight damage to, or pressure on the veins may occur. Deep-vein thrombosis

may lead to swelling of the whole leg, or it may show little outward sign of its occurrence and thus may be almost impossible to diagnose. When severe swelling is present and the leg is white and painful, the name *Phlegmasia Alba Dolens* may be used.

The most dreaded and all too common sequel to deep-vein thrombosis is pulmonary embolism, in which a piece of the thrombus breaks off and is carried in the blood to the lungs. A small piece may cause an infarct in the lung. A large piece may completely obstruct the arteries to the lungs, and if this happens the patient dies suddenly. It is largely because of the very real risk of pulmonary embolism that patients are made to get out of their beds and walk, in an attempt to prevent the formation of deep-vein thrombus.

HYPERTENSION

In hypertension, the pressure of the blood is higher than normal. It is sometimes called systemic hypertension to distinguish it from pulmonary hypertension. A patient may be said to have systemic hypertension when the arterial blood pressure recorded by the sphygmomanometer is more than 140/90 mm of mercury. The lower figure, the diastolic pressure, is the important one in assessing hypertension.

The arteries are like tubes. The pressure in these tubes depends on the heart which pushes blood in at one end, and it also depends on the arterioles which control the flow of blood out at the other end, into the capillaries (Figure 7-3). Between the two ends there is a pressure, the diastolic pressure, which is boosted every time the heart gives a systolic contraction and pumps more blood into the system. It is rather like playing the bagpipes. The piper puffs up the bag from time to time, just as the heart does with its systolic contractions, to give a boost of pressure. At the other end of the bag, there is a controlled loss of pressure through the chanter and the pipes, which in this analogy resemble the arterioles.

The arterioles are small vessels, not much more than one hundredth of a millimetre in diameter. Although they are small, there are many of them, and they have muscle in their walls which can expand or contract to allow more or less blood to pass through. If the arterioles are wide open, there is little resistance to

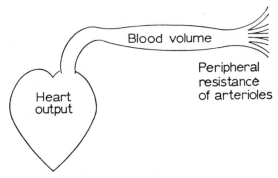

FIG. 7-3 The three components of blood pressure

the flow of blood, but if they contract, the resistance rises, and rises very steeply. In fact, if an arteriole contracts to half its former diameter, the resistance is increased not twice but sixteen times, and thus the resistance of the arterioles is very important in controlling the blood pressure.

The state of the arterioles is the key factor in the blood pressure, and there are three main systems which control the arterioles: the kidneys, the adrenals and the sympathetic nervous system.

The flow of blood through the kidneys may be reduced, either by narrowing of the renal arteries by atherosclerosis or by diseases which damage the kidney, such as pyelonephritis, which damages the arteries within the kidney. .The kidney reacts to any such reduction of blood flow by making a chemical called *Renin*, which passes into the blood. Renin combines with a protein in the blood to form *Angiotensin* and this has a direct and powerful constricting effect on the walls of the arterioles, which raises th. blood pressure.

The second organ concerned with the control of blood pressure is the adrenal gland, and both the medulla and the cortex of the adrenal are involved. The medulla secretes two hormones into the blood, adrenalin and noradrenalin, both of which stimulate the arterioles to contract.

A hormone from the outer part of the adrenal gland, the cortex, also affects the blood pressure. This is aldosterone, which has no action on the arterioles, but does tend to raise the blood pressure by encouraging the retention of sodium and water in the body. The increased water content swells the volume of the blood and raises the blood pressure.

The adrenal cortex is controlled by the hormones secreted by the pituitary gland, and thus disorders of the pituitary may also affect the blood pressure.

The third system controlling the blood pressure starts with the pressure receptors in the arch of the aorta and in the carotid arteries. These are sensitive nerve endings in the walls of these arteries which can measure the blood pressure. They are connected by nerves to the brain, and from there via the sympathetic nervous system to the arterioles (Figure 7-4).

'Biofeedback' machines are gadgets which continuously measure the blood pressure, and show flashing lights or other signals when the blood pressure falls. By using such machines, some people can learn to control and lower their blood pressure themselves. The conscious mind may therefore play a part in the normal control of blood pressure, and mental stress could perhaps be a factor contributing to hypertension in some people.

In every patient with hypertension it is important to look for a cause but a cause is found only in one case out of every ten patients. The causes found are shown below:

(1) *Kidney*—Obstructions of the renal artery, or diseases damaging the kidney and its vessels such as pyelonephritis.

(2) *Adrenal*—Medulla: tumour (Phaeochromocytoma). Cortex: excessive aldosterone production, sometimes due to pituitary disorders.

(3) *Brain*—Occasionally a rapidly expanding brain tumour.

In the other nine cases out of ten, no specific cause is found. It is probable that

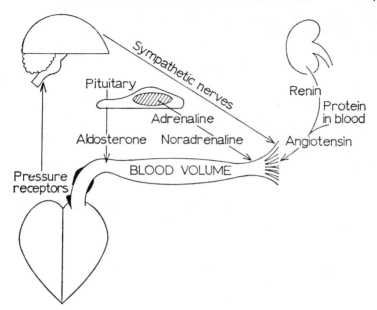

FIG. 7-4 The factors which control the three components of blood pressure

in some of these cases the 'setting' of one of the various mechanisms controlling the blood pressure is higher than normal, just as the 'setting' of a central heating thermostat may be higher than normal. Some of these patients may have inherited a tendency to hypertension from their parents. The term Essential Hypertension is used for these cases when no cause for the hypertension can be found.

In hypertension, pathological changes occur in the arterioles. The contraction of the muscle fibres in the walls of the arterioles eventually becomes permanent as fibrous material is deposited in their walls. This fibrous material most particularly affects the arterioles in the kidneys, and may lead to further kidney damage, and a vicious circle is set up by further secretions of renin from the kidney.

Other pathological changes occur in the heart and in the large arteries. The muscle of the left ventricle of the heart has to work harder to maintain the blood flow to the various organs and it responds by becoming thicker. Hypertension is a potent factor in the production of atherosclerosis, and thus the arteries are also changed in hypertension. The berry aneurysms on the cerebral arteries have already been mentioned (page 75). They are particularly liable to form in patients with hypertension, and may burst and cause a cerebral haemorrhage. The effects of hypertension are therefore widespread, as arterioles and arteries, and heart, kidneys and brain may all be affected.

Surprisingly, many people live with these changes for many years, and death when it does come may be due to some entirely unconnected cause. Of the patients that do die of the effects of hypertension, 60 per cent die of heart failure, as the left ventricle can no longer cope with its increased workload, 30 per cent die of kidney failure and 10 per cent die of thrombosis or haemorrhage of the cerebral arteries.

Malignant hypertension, as the name suggests, is a severe form of hypertension. Some people think it is a separate disease. It tends to affect men about 40 years old, and the diastolic pressure is very high, over 120 mm of mercury. Fibrin is deposited in the walls of the arterioles, and the patients suffer severe kidney damage, with numerous small haemorrhages and sometimes with blood in the urine. The haemorrhages can be seen in the eyes through an ophthalmoscope, and they also develop swelling of the optic cup, a condition called *papilloedema*. Fortunately malignant hypertension is not common. Death from kidney failure usually occurs within a year from the onset of malignant hypertension in untreated cases.

Hypertension occurs in two other conditions, acute glomerulonephritis and pre-eclamptic toxaemia of pregnancy. These conditions however do not usually last long enough for the hypertension to become permanent.

8 *DISEASES OF THE HEART*

CORONARY ARTERY DISEASE
Angina Pectoris

Diffuse Myocardial Fibrosis

Coronary Artery Thrombosis and Myocardial Infarct

MYOPATHIES

HYPERTENSIVE HEART DISEASE

DISEASES PRINCIPALLY AFFECTING THE VALVES OF THE HEART
General Features

Congenital Valve Diseases

Rheumatic Fever and Rheumatic Heart Disease

Subacute Bacterial Endocarditis

Calcific Aortic Stenosis

PERICARDITIS

TUMOURS

CORONARY ARTERY DISEASE

In the previous chapter, we discussed the development of plaques of atheroma in the walls of arteries. This process occurs in the coronary arteries, and all too frequently proves fatal, due to thrombus development on a plaque. Heart disease kills some 200 000 people each year in the United Kingdom and a million a year in the United States, more than all the forms of cancer put together, and four out of every five of these deaths are due to coronary artery disease.

Angina Pectoris

If the coronary arteries are narrowed by plaques of atheroma, the blood supply to the heart muscle may be reduced to a level that is adequate only at rest. The ischaemia of the myocardium may result in angina pectoris, or in diffuse myocardial fibrosis or both.

Angina pectoris is the severe and limiting chest pain that occurs when the heart muscle is made to do more pumping work than its own blood supply will allow. The cramp-like pain passes off again if the patient rests and allows the blood supply to catch up with the demand, and there may be no permanent damage to the heart muscle.

Diffuse Myocardial Fibrosis

Diffuse myocardial fibrosis is the name for the small scars scattered through the heart muscle which may accumulate through the years, each due to a small work overload of the moderately ischaemic heart muscle. The gradual replacement of heart muscle by scar tissue may eventually cause congestive cardiac failure (see Chapter 4), but often these patients manage to live a long, though somewhat limited, life.

Coronary Artery Thrombosis and Myocardial Infarct

It is thrombosis of one of the coronary arteries that is the major killer. It causes infarction of part of the myocardium (Figure 8-1).

The cells in the affected area of the myocardium die, and so do any cells of the impulse-conducting system that may be involved. An infarct of the myocardium has the typical form of an infarct. The centre is composed of dead myocardial cells, together with red blood cells that escape from the small blood vessels. The area of dead muscle is soft and flabby and completely incapable of contracting. Gradually the dead area loses its normal brown colour, and over a few days it goes soft and yellow, and it becomes surrounded by a red ring of inflammatory reaction around the edges. If the patient manages to survive, the dead cells slowly dissolve away and are replaced, over the next few months, by fibrous scar tissue.

As the cells die and dissolve away, various enzymes are released into the blood. High enzyme levels can be detected by chemical tests on the serum. The enzymes particularly concerned are called serum glutamic oxalate transaminase, serum hydroxybutyrate dehydrogenase and creatinine phosphokinase (usually abbreviated to SGOT, SHBD and CPK_1).

The typical coronary patient suffers a sudden severe constricting pain in the chest under the sternum, and feels faint and giddy. He is pale, cold and sweaty and may have a blue face. The important observations are the pulse, blood pressure and urine output if any. The pulse is thin, thready, weak and often irregular. This is an example of cardiac or central shock and the blood pressure may be so low as to be unrecordable. About a third of all coronary patients die within an hour or so of the attack, before anything can possibly be done for them. Note that though we may refer to them as coronary patients, it is really the resulting infarcts that kill them.

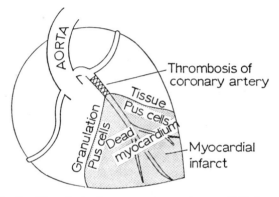

FIG. 8-1 Thrombosis of a coronary artery and myocardial infarct

About a third of them survive long enough to get to hospital. They require careful monitoring, particularly of the blood pressure and of the electrocardiographic trace. This records the electrical changes that are normally conducted through the heart muscle to cause it to contract regularly. An infarct may upset this system, either by direct damage to the cells that conduct the electrical impulses, or because electrical changes in the dying muscle cells may themselves act as a stimulus to the nearby muscle cells, and cause them to contract irregularly. These out of place, or ectopic foci of electrical stimulation may give rise to various arrhythmias, the most feared of which is known as ventricular fibrillation.

The blood pressure is monitored because if it falls too low for too long, the tubules of the kidney may suffer irreparable damage, and parts of the brain may be similarly damaged.

About half of the patients admitted to hospital die as a result of hypotension or arrhythmias. The other half often require treatment for arrhythmias or hypotension, but they survive.

The remaining third or more of all coronary patients survive without such treatment. They require complete rest for several weeks, during which time the dead heart muscle is replaced by a tough fibrous scar. The scar cannot contract like muscle, but it serves as a patch, rather like the darning of a hole in a sock.

Occasionally the patch bulges outwards to form an aneurysm, and occasionally it may rupture with catastrophic results.

For the survivors, gentle but steady exercise is required. This may have little effect on the arteries that are already damaged by atherosclerosis, but it does help to prevent the damage getting worse. It also encourages any collateral blood supply to increase, such as from the other coronary artery. Thirdly it boosts the patient's morale. It prevents him from regarding himself as a complete cardiac cripple.

MYOPATHIES

The myopathies are other diseases that damage the myocardium. They are rare, but we should just mention myopathies due to toxins such as the exotoxin released by diphtheria bacteria, myopathies due to Coxsackie viruses in children, and myopathies due to generalised metabolic diseases such as amyloidosis.

HYPERTENSIVE HEART DISEASE

The topic of hypertension has been discussed in the previous chapter, and it is only necessary here to add one or two remarks about the changes that occur in the heart.

The chamber of the heart that pumps blood round the body is the left ventricle. In hypertension, the resistance against which it pumps is increased. To maintain an adequate blood flow, the muscle cells in the wall of the left ventricle enlarge, and the wall of the left ventricle becomes much thicker than usual. This is called left ventricular hypertrophy, and it can be considered as a form of compensation for the extra work load required of it. The hypertrophy is usually enough to cope with the extra work load for a long time, but eventually further increase of the resistance of the arterioles may outstrip the capacity of the heart to compensate. This is called decompensation, and presents as congestive cardiac failure. It is thus when decompensation occurs that hypertensive heart disease is most obvious.

DISEASES PRINCIPALLY AFFECTING THE VALVES OF THE HEART
General Features

Each of the four chambers of the heart expels its blood through a valve (Figure 8-2). Each valve is constructed like a pair of doors that can open outwards but not inwards, so that blood can shoot out of the doors but cannot get back in again. (Actually the tricuspid, pulmonary and aortic valves each have three of these flaps.) In some valve diseases, the doors do not open properly, a condition called stenosis, and the chamber of the heart must work very hard to force the blood out. In other cases, the valve flaps will not close properly and this is called incompetence of the valve. In this case, the blood that has been expelled tends to come back into the chamber after each contraction, and so the chamber has to push a greater volume of blood out with each stroke to maintain an adequate circulation. In some cases, the valve becomes stuck in the half-open position and it is both stenosed and incompetent at the same time.

Such valvular defects may often be heard through the stethoscope. Then the normal heart sounds which have been likened to LUBB-DUPP, LUBB-DUPP may be

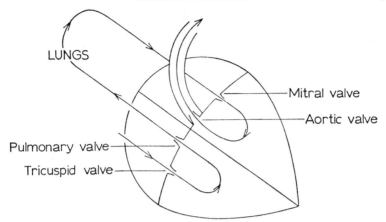

FIG. 8-2 The heart valves in the normal circulation

altered, and extra sounds or murmurs may be heard, such as LUBB-murmur-DUPP, LUBB-murmur-DUPP.

In valve diseases, the chamber concerned is usually capable of considerable hypertrophy to compensate for this defect (Figure 8-3). But eventually, the work required may exceed the capacity for hypertrophy. Decompensation occurs, and these patients typically die at the age of about 35 or 40 after some years of increasing congestive cardiac failure.

Congenital Valve Diseases

About three out of every thousand children are born with some form of congenital cardiac abnormality. There are many forms of abnormality and they will not be discussed in detail here. A few cases are due to exposure of the mother during the

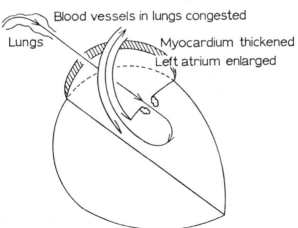

FIG. 8-3 Mitral stenosis—an example of valve disease

early months of pregnancy to rubella (German measles), or to cortisone or the now-abolished drug, thalidomide. In most cases, no cause is known.

The effects of these abnormalities are many and various. Some of them can be compensated for by myocardial hypertrophy, but most of them put a load on the myocardium that is eventually fatal unless corrected by operation.

Rheumatic Fever and Rheumatic Heart Disease

Rheumatic fever is an acute fever which occurs mainly in children and adolescents. It follows, in a few people, about three weeks after an infection of the throat by certain strains of streptococci. Most individuals develop antibodies which destroy the capsules of such streptococci and they recover from the sore throat without further ado, but in a few people rheumatic fever follows the infection.

There is a substance in the capsules of some streptococci which is chemically very similar to a substance in human connective tissue. It may be that in rheumatic fever patients, the antibodies developed against the streptococci also react with the connective tissue substance. Rheumatic fever patients have an acute fever, with aches and pains flitting from one joint to another, and with inflammation in the joints, the muscles, the pericardium, the myocardium and the heart valves. Very occasionally the inflammation of the myocardium and pericardium is severe enough to be fatal. But in nearly all cases, the inflammation subsides leaving only a few traces of fibrosis. It is only the valve damage that remains.

On the surface of the valves, small firm nodules of fibrin form and these are called vegetations. They form particularly along the lines where the edges of the valves come together and they cause the valve to be either stenosed, or incompetent, or both. The mitral valve is the most commonly affected.

The left atrium may be able to compensate for the defective valve for some years, but unless the valve is replaced surgically, decompensation is liable to occur. The patient may survive for some years as a cardiac cripple before premature death due to heart failure. It is thus the subsequent valve damage that is the main problem in Rheumatic Heart Disease.

Subacute Bacterial Endocarditis

An organism called *Streptococcus viridans* is present in most bad teeth. When such a tooth is extracted, it is almost inevitable for a shower of these usually harmless bacteria to enter the bloodstream. In most people, the bacteria are phagocytosed in about half an hour, and they do no damage, but heart valves deformed by congenital heart disease or by rheumatic heart disease seem to provide particularly suitable sites for these bacteria to grow and multiply, and they are very difficult to eradicate. For this reason, patients with congenital or rheumatic valve disease require special antibiotic protection every time they have a tooth extracted.

Another organism that is sometimes responsible is *Streptococcus faecalis*, which is normally a harmless inhabitant of the gut. The bacteria form large, soft, crumbly vegetations on the valves which look rather like cornflakes.

Small fragments of these vegetations may brush off from time to time and form septic emboli. They may lodge almost anywhere in the body, and develop into abscesses, in the brain for instance, or they may cause mycotic aneurysms. It may be necessary to take repeated blood specimens for culture before the presence of these clumps of bacteria in the blood can be demonstrated.

The disease is nearly always subacute: that is to say that the onset is not acute but insidious. It cannot be called chronic because, if untreated, the patient will die before a chronic state is reached.

Calcific Aortic Stenosis
This fourth and last form of valve disease is common in elderly people. In this condition, the aortic valve becomes stiff and calcified, usually causing a combination of stenosis and incompetence. No one knows what causes it, though some cases may be due to long-previous rheumatic heart disease.

PERICARDITIS
As the name implies, this is an inflammation of the pericardium, the tough bag which surrounds the heart and which normally contains only about a teaspoonful of watery lubricating fluid between it and the heart.

The pericardium may be involved by disease spreading from elsewhere, such as by spread of infection or tumour from the lung, or it may be involved in some condition that affects the whole body, such as uraemia. It is never, or almost never, the primary site of disease.

The importance of pericarditis is that the amount of fluid in the pericardium may be increased, or the lining of the pericardium may be swollen by inflammation. Either of these changes may embarrass the pumping action of the heart, and sometimes this is fatal.

Occasionally an infarct in the heart may cause bleeding into the pericardial sac, and the heart may be unable to pump adequately due to the pressure of the blood in the sac outside it. This condition, *cardiac tamponade*, is an uncommon cause of central shock.

TUMOURS
Primary tumours of the heart are almost unknown, and secondary tumour deposits in the heart are also uncommon.

9 DISEASES OF THE BLOOD AND LYMPH NODES

RED BLOOD CELLS
Anaemia

Iron Deficiency Anaemia

Maturation Factor Deficiency
Vitamin B_{12} Deficiency—Pernicious Anaemia
Folic Acid Deficiency
Other Causes of Megaloblastic Anaemia

Haemolytic Anaemia
Haemochromatosis
Transfusion Haemosiderosis
Malaria

Anaemias Due to Diseases Affecting the Bone Marrow

Polycythaemia

WHITE BLOOD CELLS
Leucopenia

Leucocytosis

Leukaemia

Myelofibrosis

Leukaemoid Reaction

Myelomatosis

LYMPH NODES
Sarcoidosis

Tumours of Lymph Nodes
Hodgkin's Disease
Other Tumours of Lymph Nodes

Infectious Mononucleosis

The blood cells in men occupy 42-52 per cent of the volume of the blood, in women, about 5 per cent less. It is with the cells rather than the fluid fraction of the blood that we are here concerned. The most numerous of the cells are the red blood cells, of which there are about 1000 for every white blood cell.

Of the white blood cells, the polymorphonuclear leucocytes are concerned with ingesting and dissolving dead tissue cells and bacteria. Other kinds of white blood cells, principally the lymphocytes, are the cells of cellular immunity. The lymphocytes are formed mainly in the lymph nodes, whereas the polymorphs and the red blood cells are formed in the bone marrow.

Any change in the bone marrow may affect the red cells and the white cells, together with the blood platelets which are also formed in the marrow. The bone marrow is central to any discussion of diseases of the blood cells, and examination of the bone marrow cells is often necessary in investigation of diseases of the blood cells.

RED BLOOD CELLS
Anaemia
Anaemia is a deficiency of haemoglobin, and this means a deficiency of the red blood cells which consist almost entirely of haemoglobin. A deficiency of haemoglobin causes a deficient oxygen supply to all parts of the body. There is weakness and fatigue. The mucous membranes, tongue and lips are pale. The heart has a high output, with a rapid pulse rate, in an attempt to compensate for the oxygen deficit. Decompensation may eventually occur and lead to congestive cardiac failure. There is shortness of breath, and there may be headache or dizziness. In some cases of long-standing anaemia, the heart muscle may atrophy, and this is an indication of the severe effects which may result from a persistently poor oxygen supply.

Anaemia may be due to a shortage of iron or of the maturation factors required for making blood cells. It may be due to abnormal destruction of red blood cells (haemolysis) or it may be due to diseases affecting the bone marrow.

Iron Deficiency Anaemia
Normally, red blood cells survive in the blood for about 100-120 days, after which time they are destroyed, mainly in the spleen. The iron they contain is kept in the body to be used to make new blood cells. However, if blood is lost from the body by bleeding, the iron is also lost, and if this loss is greater than the iron intake in foods such as meat and vegetables, iron deficiency occurs, and iron deficiency is by far the commonest cause of anaemia.

In infants, there is normally enough iron in their bodies at birth to last them during the first six months of life, but after that they may become anaemic if their diet still consists of little but milk, as milk contains no iron.

In women, there are two particular processes which commonly cause anaemia. These are the blood losses that occur at the menstrual periods, and the the extra quantity of iron needed for the foetus and placenta and for the mother herself, during pregnancy.

Apart from the obvious loss of blood due to injury, there may be a hidden or occult loss of blood, and this may occur in men, women or children. The alimentary tract is where this commonly occurs. The blood loss may occur in oesophagitis or oesophageal varices, in the stomach in peptic ulcer or carcinoma or with excess aspirin intake, and in the intestines due to hookworm (ankylostomiasis), carcinoma, ulcerative colitis or piles. A most valuable investigation in such cases is the demonstration of blood in the faeces. Until recently, the Haematest method was the most widely used, but this has been withdrawn on account of the alleged carcinogenic action of one of the reagents. The other test methods available are less satisfactory.

Any of these causes may create an iron deficiency, and since iron is an important constituent of haemoglobin, a deficiency of iron means that the amount of haemoglobin in the red blood cells is reduced. The red blood cells are small (microcytic) and pale (hypochromic) and they are in short supply. The red blood cells are not the only cells affected by iron deficiency. There is often a spoon-shaped hollow in the fingernails (*koilonychia*), a loss of papillae of the tongue (*atrophic glossitis*) and there may also be vague abdominal discomfort, as well as all the general features of anaemia described previously.

Maturation Factor Deficiency

Vitamin B_{12} (cyanocobalamin) and folic acid are chemical substances which are referred to as maturation factors. If there is a deficiency of either of them, the blood-forming cells of the bone marrow can only mature into red cells very slowly. The cells in the marrow tend to become larger and larger, accumulating more and more haemoglobin before they eventually mature into red blood cells. The large marrow cells can be seen down the microscope and are called megaloblasts, and the resulting anaemia is called a *megaloblastic anaemia*.

The red blood cells that are eventually released into the circulation are also big and they are called *macrocytes*. They may also be very varied in shape (poikilocytosis) and in size (anisocytosis).

The other kinds of cell in the bone marrow may also be affected, resulting in a *pancytopenia*; that is a deficiency of polymorphs and blood platelets as well as anaemia.

VITAMIN B_{12} DEFICIENCY—PERNICIOUS ANAEMIA (Also called Addisonian Anaemia)
A substance called the *intrinsic factor* is made by the stomach gland cells and is present in normal gastric juice. In the absence of intrinsic factor in the stomach juice, vitamin B_{12} from the food cannot be absorbed further down in the intestine, and a megaloblastic anaemia called Pernicious Anaemia is the result.

The cause of intrinsic factor deficiency is a form of atrophic gastritis, in which the cells that normally form intrinsic factor, which are also the cells which make hydrochloric acid, are lost. Pernicious anaemia is always associated with a complete absence of stomach acid (achlorhydria). The precise cause of the loss of these cells is not known, but it appears that for some unknown reason the body forms anti-bodies which destroy the cells, and that this is an auto-immune process.

The disease affects people over 40, mainly women. Apart from the general effects of anaemia previously mentioned, such as fatigue, there are particular changes in pernicious anaemia such as a smooth tongue, sometimes with fissures running across it like a map ('geographical glossitis'), and a lemon-yellow tinge to the eyeballs. Deficiency of vitamin B_{12} may also cause a peripheral neuritis with tingling and loss of sensation of the hands and feet. In a few cases, there may be a condition called *Subacute Combined Degeneration of the Spinal Cord*, which shows as unsteadiness in walking. One other feature which should be mentioned is that pernicious anaemia patients, even after satisfactory treatment by injections of vitamin B_{12}, have three times the normal risk of developing carcinoma of the stomach.

FOLIC ACID DEFICIENCY

The absorption of folic acid is seldom impaired . Any deficiency is due to an inade-quate intake of the foods which contain folic acid, such as uncooked green vege-tables, lettuces and the like. The commonest time for a deficiency to become apparent is during pregnancy, when more folic acid than normal is required.

OTHER CAUSES OF MEGALOBLASTIC ANAEMIA

Deficiencies of vitamin B_{12} or folic acid, or sometimes of both together, may occasionally occur in malabsorption, after gastrectomy, or in patients being treated with Phenytoin or Primidone for epilepsy.

Haemolytic Anaemia   *Increased RBC destruction .*

In haemolytic anaemias, the red blood cells do not survive in the circulation for the usual 100 days or so but are destroyed much earlier. Sometimes the bone marrow can compensate for this by making more red cells, but sometimes the rate of destruction is so high that the bone marrow compensate is inadequate, and then anaemia develops and may be severe. The large amount of pigment liberated from the broken-down red cells may be seen as jaundice, which may be described as *Acholuric* jaundice, to indicate that no blood pigments are present in the urine.

There is a multiplicity of possible causes for haemolytic anaemias. Sometimes the red blood cells are destroyed prematurely because they are abnormally formed, and this happens in a condition called congenital spherocytosis, and in another hereditary condition called sickle cell anaemia. There is also a group of hereditary conditions called the haemoglobinopathies, in which the chemical composition of the haemoglobin is slightly different from normal, and the red cells in this condition suffer the same fate. Another cause of abnormal red cell formation has already been mentioned, and that is the megaloblastic anaemias.

The red blood cells may also be destroyed due to some change occurring to them in the circulation, such as infestation with malarial parasites, or damage by some drug such as Phenacetin. In other cases, for some unknown reason, the body develops an immune response to its own red blood cells, either by forming antibodies or by the development of a cellular immunity (auto-immune haemolytic anaemia).

The haemolytic anaemias are important, though they are not common. Blood transfusion is often required, especially in treatment of the acute crises of haemolysis which may occur from time to time. Some of the patients may require 500 or more units of blood over the years, and this has its own dangers as they run a serious risk of developing liver damage due to serum hepatitis from infected donor blood. They are also liable to damage from the accumulation in the liver of large amounts of iron from the haemolysed cells, a condition called *haemosiderosis*.

HAEMOCHROMATOSIS

This rare disease is mentioned here as it concerns the absorption of iron. In haemo-chromatosis, there is excessive absorption of iron from the food, and over the years an enormous quantity of iron accumulates in the body. The disease has an hereditary tendency. It is probably an inborn error of metabolism, a genetic defect of the iron absorption mechanism.

Haemochromatosis affects men, usually in their late middle age. Women are very seldom affected, perhaps because the normal menstrual loss of iron tends to balance any excessive absorption that they may have. The accumulation of vast amounts of iron in the body causes cirrhosis of the liver, atrophy of the pancreas, diabetes mellitus, and pigmentation of the skin. The older name for haemochromatosis was bronzed diabetes. The patients may die of heart or liver failure.

TRANSFUSION HAEMOSIDEROSIS

Patients with haemolytic anaemia may require hundreds of units of transfused blood, to make up for the excessive breakdown of their red blood cells. Over the years, they may accumulate large amounts of iron in their bodies, but for some unknown reason, the iron derived from blood breakdown only occasionally leads to the liver or other damage seen in haemochromatosis.

MALARIA

Malaria is no longer present in Great Britain, but it is still numerically one of the most important of the world's diseases. The four types of *Plasmodium* parasite cause somewhat differing patterns of the disease. All four types are carried by mosquitoes. The Plasmodia are transmitted when the mosquito bites, and they infect the blood cells and liver and cause anaemia. The spleen may be much enlarged, partly due to its haemolytic activity, and it may even rupture. In many cases, the infection becomes chronic, but if the organism is of the type known as *Plasmodium falci-parum*, there is a severe fever and many small blood vessels become plugged by parasitised blood cells. The brain is particularly affected, together with the heart and kidneys, and death is not uncommon, especially in young children.

Anaemias Due to Diseases Affecting the Bone Marrow

The marrow may be directly affected by various poisons such as anti-tuberculous drugs, anti-thyroid drugs and anti-tumour drugs or X-rays. The activity of the marrow cells is depressed and the resulting anaemia is called an *aplastic anaemia.* Leukaemia has a similar effect and anaemia is a constant feature of this disease. Sometimes the production of polymorphs and blood platelets is affected, as well as the red cells, resulting in the multiple deficiency called *pancytopenia.*

A similar depression of bone marrow activity may also be seen as a secondary phenomenon associated with diseases of other parts of the body. Common causes of this are severe infections such as widespread tuberculosis, or renal failure, disseminated lupus erythematosus, and carcinomatosis.

Polycythaemia
This is an uncommon condition in which an excess of red cells is produced, and the volume of red cells in the blood is raised well above the normal upper level of 52 per cent. The cause is unknown, but the effect is that the viscosity of the blood is increased, and thrombosis commonly occurs. The patients are usually men of late middle age, and they are often hypertensive. They may suffer from thrombotic or sometimes haemorrhagic incidents, often involving the brain.

WHITE BLOOD CELLS
Leucopenia
A deficiency of white blood cells may occur in any of the diseases previously mentioned which affect the bone marrow. *Agranulocytosis* is a specific deficiency of the granulocytic white cells. These are principally the polymorphs, the main function of which is to destroy bacteria. Infections, such as sore throats, are common in this deficiency, and may progress to fatal pneumonias. Drugs such as Chloramphenicol and Thiouracil have been responsible in some cases.

Leucocytosis
Increased numbers of different kinds of white cells in the blood are common in infections, injuries, myocardial infarcts and many other diseases. The eosinophilic white cells are particularly increased in allergic conditions and in diseases due to parasites. The lymphocytes are increased in almost every infection in children, especially whooping cough, and in adults they are increased in virus diseases such as influenza and also in glandular fever.

Leukaemia
Leukaemia, despite the publicity, is fortunately an uncommon condition, but an important one. It is a neoplastic disease of the bone marrow cells, which results in the production of large numbers of abnormal white blood cells. Different varieties of leukaemia are recognised, but they all have various features in common: *Anaemia* is nearly always present, and reduction in the numbers of the blood platelets (thrombocytopenia) is common, and this may be the cause of the *haemorrhages* and/or *thromboses* which are commonly seen. The other very frequent occurrence is *infection*, due probably to the fact that the leukaemic cells are abnormal not only in form but also in function.

Leukaemia is a form of cancer in which there is an uncontrolled proliferation of white blood cells, but it differs from most other forms of cancer in that it is a diffuse process which only very occasionally produces any lump or tumour. In aleukaemic leukaemia, the bone marrow cells are abnormal and show all the features of leukaemia, but no abnormal cells are present in the circulating blood. Usually aleukaemic leukaemia progresses to fully developed leukaemia, and leukaemic cells eventually appear in the blood.

The causation and also the immunotherapy of leukaemia are discussed in Chapter 5.

Myelofibrosis

In this uncommon condition, fibre-making cells in the bone marrow proliferate, and much of the blood-forming marrow is replaced by fibrous tissue. In many cases, blood-forming tissue develops in the liver and spleen, and these organs become much enlarged. No one knows what causes myelofibrosis. Some cases eventually go on to develop leukaemia.

Leukaemoid Reaction

Primitive white cells from the bone marrow may be found in the blood in some severe infections, in acute haemolysis or with secondary tumour deposits in the marrow, and this appearance is called a leukaemoid reaction. Examination of a specimen of bone marrow is sometimes required to distinguish between it and leukaemia.

Myelomatosis

Myelomatosis is a malignant disease in which numerous tumours develop in the bone marrow, formed of abnormal plasma cells. The cells proliferate and erode the adjacent bone and X-ray examination shows numerous circular cavities in the bone. The function of normal plasma cells is to make antibodies and the abnormal plasma cells in myelomatosis make abnormal antibodies in large quantities, and these can nearly always be detected in the blood serum, and often also in the urine (see also Chapter 3).

LYMPH NODES

The 'glands' in the neck which are commonly present in patients with sore throats are lymph nodes which are enlarged by a proliferation of their cells in reaction to bacteria or bacterial substances in the lymph. There are very few diseases in which the lymph nodes are not involved in one way or another, and it is often useful to biopsy a lymph node for microscopic examination to determine what kind of disease is present. One disease in which the lymph nodes are nearly always involved is Sarcoidosis.

Sarcoidosis

Sarcoidosis is an uncommon disease. The cause is unknown, although the changes seen down the microscope resemble the granulomas of tuberculosis. It has been found that pine pollen can induce similar microscopic changes, and so can various other agents, but there is no proof that the tuberculosis bacillus, or pine pollen, or any other agent is in fact responsible.

The lymph nodes are nearly always affected in sarcoidosis, with granulomas or fibrosis. The other organs that may be involved include the lungs, the heart, the salivary glands, the eyes and the skin. The curious features of the disease include increased levels of globulins and calcium in the blood, and changes of skin reactivity to antigens. The skin reaction to tuberculin protein is depressed or absent, but there may be a positive reaction to a test injection of human sarcoid tissue extract (the Kveim test). The disease runs an indolent course, and is seldom fatal, unless the heart or lungs are severely affected.

Tumours of Lymph Nodes

A characteristic of cancer arising in lymph nodes is that it tends to develop in several lymph nodes at once, with a multifocal origin, and in this respect it shows some similarity to leukaemias. But the affected lymph nodes, unlike leukaemia, develop into nodules and lumps of tumour tissue and the process slowly spreads to involve other groups of lymph nodes.

The distinction between the varieties of lymph node tumour depends largely on the microscopic appearances, which need not concern us, but one or two of the features of each can be briefly mentioned.

HODGKIN'S DISEASE

Hodgkin's disease is the commonest of the lymph node tumours, and it quite often shows first as an enlargement of the lymph nodes in one side of the neck. Later, the lymph nodes in the chest or abdomen may be involved. The lymph nodes may be enlarged up to 10 cm in diameter, and the massive lymph node enlargement may cause death, due to the effects of pressure or obstruction on vital organs.

It is not perhaps surprising, as it is the lymph nodes that are involved, that patients with Hodgkin's disease frequently also have disturbances of their immune defence mechanism, and some of these patients succumb eventually to infections, often by relatively innocuous organisms such as *Candida albicans* (Monilia or Thrush).

Hodgkin's disease is one variety of cancer which can sometimes be completely cured by heavy doses of radiotherapy or combinations of drugs.

OTHER TUMOURS OF LYMPH NODES

The other tumours of lymph nodes present a range from the follicular lymphomas of low malignancy, through lymphosarcomas to reticulum cell sarcomas in which the average time from diagnosis to death is only a year or so, but these tumours are very unpredictable in their behaviour, and some patients survive very much longer than a year.

Infectious Mononucleosis (Glandular fever)

This disease is not a cancer. It is almost certainly an infection due to a virus, but the virus responsible has not been identified. There is some evidence that it is spread by kissing. It affects young adults, with general malaise and depression, a low-grade fever, sore throat and enlargement of the lymph nodes and spleen. Sometimes the liver is also involved. The involvement of the lymph nodes may perhaps be responsible for two changes seen in the peripheral blood. One is the appearance in the blood of rather primitive lymphocytes, and the other is the development of curious antibodies which can be demonstrated by the Paul-Bunnell laboratory test.

10 *DISEASES OF THE RESPIRATORY TRACT*

INFECTIONS
The Common Cold

Tonsillitis, Pharyngitis, Laryngitis, Tracheitis and Otitis Media

Acute Bronchitis and Bronchopneumonia

Lobar Pneumonia and Pleurisy

Empyema

Primary Atypical Pneumonia

Tuberculosis
Primary Infection
Re-infection

CHRONIC BRONCHITIS
Emphysema

Bronchial Asthma

Pneumoconiosis

Tumours of the Upper Respiratory Tract

Carcinoma of the Bronchus (Bronchogenic Carcinoma)

Bronchiectasis

Pneumothorax

Hydrothorax

It has been estimated that the lungs have a surface area of 90 square metres, the same area as about 140 double pages of an average newspaper. At rest, we expose this surface to about 500 ml of air with each breath we take, and each ml of air may contain between 1 and 100 or more bacteria, not to mention traces of noxious gases and dust particles.

Infection of the lungs is only prevented by an extremely efficient protection mechanism, the main elements of which are mucus and cilia in the bronchi, and phagocytic cells in the lung alveoli. Slimy mucus lines the air passages and this traps all but the smallest air-borne particles, and the cilia in the lining of the bronchi constantly beat and propel the mucus up towards the throat where it can be removed by coughing. The phagocytic cells in the alveoli ingest any particles that may escape the mucus trap.

INFECTIONS
The Common Cold
Several different viruses may cause the common cold, including a small group of viruses called Rhinoviruses. The viruses damage some of the epithelial cells and give rise to a mild inflammation of the lining of the nose and throat and sometimes of the eyes. There is a watery discharge, and the condition then subsides after two or three days, when a cellular immunity develops.

But, as anyone who has dealings with snotty-nosed children knows, bacterial infection frequently follows. The bacteria involved may be any of the various strains of Staphylococci, Streptococci or Pneumococci. Pus is formed and accounts for the obnoxious yellow discharge.

This process of bacterial infection following a virus infection is a common phenomenon in the respiratory tract, and we shall meet it again when we consider bronchopneumonia.

Tonsillitis, Pharyngitis, Laryngitis, Tracheitis and Otitis Media
The respiratory tract is a continuous passage without boundaries, and an infection often involves several areas at once. In each case, the lining epithelium is inflamed and pus is often present.

TONSILLITIS
Enlargement of the tonsils and of the adenoids at the back of the nose is a normal reaction to infection, and is commonplace in children. Usually the enlargement recedes when the infection passes, but occasionally it persists and it may block the opening of the Eustachian tube which runs from the middle ear to the back of the throat, and when this happens *Otitis media*, infection of the middle ear, may follow.

PHARYNGITIS
Pharyngitis is a general term for inflammation of the passages behind the nose and

mouth. Diphtheria is one of the particular diseases that may affect the pharynx. This disease would be of little consequence were it not for two features, the tendency to form a tough sheet of dead cells and bacteria, the diphtheritic 'wash-leather' membrane which may block the airway, and the production by the bacteria of powerful chemical poisons, exotoxins, which enter the blood and damage the cells of the myocardium. Either of these complications may be fatal.

Another condition that may occasionally occur is infection of the pharynx due to *agranulocytosis*, a disease of the blood in which there is a deficiency of phagocytic white blood cells. Infection of the pharynx is sometimes the first manifestation of this condition.

TRACHEITIS

Inflammation of the trachea is associated with cough, and pain just behind the collar-stud on coughing. It usually occurs together with infection higher up or lower down in the respiratory tract.

Acute Bronchitis and Bronchopneumonia

Acute bronchitis is an acute inflammation of the lining of the bronchi due to infection. Bronchopneumonia starts as acute bronchitis, but in this case the infection spreads into the lung tissue around each bronchus so that many of the bronchi contain pus, and there are numerous small areas of inflammation and infection scattered throughout both lungs.

Bronchopneumonia often starts with a virus infection, such as influenza in old people, measles in West African children, or respiratory syncytical virus in infants. Such viruses cause only relatively mild illnesses in healthy young adults, but in the very old or the very young, or if some debilitating illness is present, bacterial infection frequently follows, and the bacteria may be Staphylococci, Streptococci, Pneumococci or others. It is this secondary bacterial infection and bronchopneumonia that accounts for the large number of deaths that may occur during an influenza epidemic.

Another cause of bronchopneumonia is the aspiration of material from the stomach, that is partly digested food and gastric juice. Such material may be drawn into the air passages if the patient attempts to breathe at the same time as vomiting, an event that may occur with an unconscious patient or during recovery from an anaesthetic. The presence of such material in the bronchi produces a severe inflammation and bacterial infection invariably follows.

Bronchopneumonia is a very common development in the last hours or days before death, and some degree of bronchopneumonia is almost always present at post-mortem examination, the only exceptions being cases of sudden death such as may occur in road traffic accidents for instance.

Bronchopneumonia is very common, either by itself, or as an accompaniment to other conditions, and its most characteristic feature is its patchy distribution throughout the lungs (Figure 10-1).

Staphylococcal bronchopneumonia is sometimes distinguished by the tendency for abscesses to form in the lungs, and these may occasionally give rise to abscesses in other parts of the body, such as the brain, by bloodstream spread of the infection.

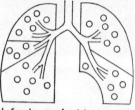 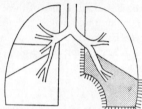

FIG. 10-1 Bronchopneumonia and lobar pneumonia—a comparison

Lobar Pneumonia and Pleurisy

This is the pneumonia which used to be responsible for the deaths of many robust young adults before penicillin became available. It still occurs, though it is seldom seen in hospital as most cases are now treated at home by their General Practitioners. The typical story is of a fit young man or woman, who develops a fever of rapid onset, a cough and a sharp pain like a knife in one side of the chest every time he or she breathes.

A Pneumococcus is almost always the causative organism. Pneumococci are present normally in the throats of about half the population, who presumably develop immunity to the strains of Pneumococci they carry. If inhaled into the lungs of a susceptible individual, an acute inflammatory response follows, and a very noticeable feature of this response is the large amount of the inflammatory exudate which contains both fluid and cells. The bacteria multiply rapidly in this fluid, and the process continues until all the air spaces in one entire lobe of the lung are completely filled with fluid, inflammatory cells and Pneumococci. The process is described as consolidation, as the normal delicate, spongy texture becomes completely airless and solid with exudate. The pleural surface of the lobe of the lung is also inflamed, and becomes covered with a shaggy layer of sticky fibrin, a condition called pleurisy.

Death sometimes occurs, but usually the patient survives either until penicillin is given, or for the five or six days which are needed for antibodies to develop to the Pneumococcus. When either penicillin or antibodies appear in the blood, the bacteria can be destroyed by phagocytic cells, and the inflammatory exudate is completely dissolved away and absorbed and the delicate spongy lung tissue reappears with little or no residual damage.

Empyema

Empyema is pus in the pleural cavity. It is due to infection spreading from the lung in lobar pneumonia or from a lung abscess due to Staphylococcal broncho-pneumonia.

Primary Atypical Pneumonia

This condition is less common than lobar pneumonia, and very much less common than bronchopneumonia. The patient slowly becomes unwell over a period of several weeks, often with very little evidence to account for it until a chest X-ray shows small patches of inflammation in the lungs, rather like bronchopneumonia. The organisms responsible, however, are not bacteria, but may be either viruses or *mycoplasma*. Mycoplasma are like very small bacteria but they lack the rigid cell wall of bacteria and they can assume varied shapes and sizes and they require special methods for culture in the laboratory. Primary atypical pneumonia is almost the only disease that mycoplasma cause in humans. The organisms are only moderately sensitive to antibiotic treatment. Most patients with primary atypical pneumonia recover, but it is often a slow recovery.

Tuberculosis

It has been estimated that about 10 per cent of the world population die of tuber-culosis. In many countries it is still the 'captain of the men of death'. In Great Britain, it is still the cause of about 2000 deaths each year, despite all our efforts at prevention.

The organism concerned is *Mycobacterium tuberculosis*. In many countries the infection may be acquired by drinking infected cow's milk, but in Great Britain the disease has been eradicated in cattle, and the only route of infection is by inhalation into the lungs of bacteria from an infected person.

PRIMARY INFECTION

When bacteria are inhaled into the lungs for the first time, they may multiply briefly, and some bacteria may be carried to the lymph nodes at the root of the lung. The cellular reaction of the body surrounds the bacteria with a small knot of cells called a tubercle, composed of phagocytic and fibrous cells, and the patient develops a cellular immunity, and destroys the organism. Thus the end result of most primary infections is some degree of cellular immunity.

In a few cases, perhaps due to some other illness, the patient does not develop an adequate degree of immunity and the tubercle bacilli multiply, and destroy some of the nearby cells. Multiplication of the bacteria together with tissue destruction may release some bacteria into a bronchus, and they may give rise to a rapidly progressive bronchopneumonia, or they may enter the blood stream and infect the whole body. Small tubercles form in all parts of the body, and they can be seen at the back of the eye. They resemble millet seeds, and this appearance gives the condition the name of *miliary tuberculosis*. Untreated, both tuberculous broncho-pneumonia and miliary tuberculosis are rapidly fatal, but appropriate antituber-culous therapy can now save most cases, though residual damage in the eyes, brain or other organs may remain.

Thus, in most cases, the primary infection causes only a small tubercle to form in the lung and another in the lymph nodes, and it leaves a lasting cellular immunity. Immunity can also be acquired by exposing a patient to a harmless form of tuberculosis bacteria which can be grown on potatoes. This form is called BCG and it produces a small tubercle in the skin of the arm where it is injected, a tubercle in the lymph nodes in the armpit and some degree of lasting cellular immunity against all varieties of tuberculosis bacteria (Figure 10-2).

TUBERCULOSIS

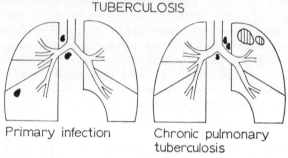

Primary infection   Chronic pulmonary
                         tuberculosis

FIG. 10-2 Pulmonary tuberculosis, primary and secondary infection

RE-INFECTION

A second or subsequent tuberculous infection is very different from the first, due to the existence of a degree of immunity following the first infection.

In most cases, there is a prompt destruction by the immune cells of any bacteria that may be inhaled, and the only evidence of infection is a very small residual scar in the lung.

In some cases, however, the degree of immunity is less effective. Inflammatory and fibrous cells move towards the bacteria, but the cells are ineffective and die without destroying the bacteria. The dead cells accumulate and form a soft cheesy material in a process called *caseation*. The fibrous cells form a wall of fibrous tissue around the area of dead cells and bacteria, to form a fibro-caseous lesion typical of tuberculosis.

A situation thus develops in which the ability of the bacteria to multiply, damage tissue cells and cause caseation is balanced by the ability of the body to produce inflammatory cells and fibrous tissues. This is an example of chronic inflammation, in which inflammation and repair continue indefinitely as the cause cannot be removed. The aim of sanatorium treatment for tuberculosis was to improve the patient's general state of health and his level of immunity so that this balance was upset in the patient's favour. The same aim is still pursued, but antituberculous drugs are now available and they are effective against all but a few resistant strains of tuberculosis.

Occasionally the Mycobacteria may spread via the bloodstream to infect distant sites such as the vertebrae or the kidneys, or form cold abscesses elsewhere. A cold abscess is so called because the outside of it consists of fibrous tissue and shows little active inflammation.

CHRONIC BRONCHITIS

In chronic bronchitis, there is a persistent over-production of watery mucus by the glands lining the bronchi, which can only be removed by persistent coughing. Microscopic examination shows that there is a big increase in the number of mucus-producing glands in the bronchi of chronic bronchitics. Other changes seen are dilatation of the bronchi and fibrous thickening of their walls.

The disease is common in Great Britain, particularly among men. When still young, they start to cough, especially on first getting up in the morning, during the winter. As the disease progresses, they need to cough more and more, all through the day, in summer as well as in winter, and most of the time it is watery mucus that is produced.

The disease is often described as though it were the result of previous infections, and doubtless this is sometimes the case, but there are other patients who develop chronic bronchitis but who have little or no history of previous infections. The disease is particularly common in industrial regions, and there is no doubt that tobacco smoke, dust and atmospheric pollution by sulphurous fumes play a large part in producing this serious and debilitating disease. Damp, cold, a hereditary tendency and various allergies to particular inhaled substances may also play a part.

The presence of mucus in the bronchi makes it difficult to remove bacteria, and bacterial infections are common complications of chronic bronchitis, particularly in the winter months. Such infections occur as acute exacerbations of the disease, and the organisms commonly responsible for them are Haemophilus influenzae and Pneumococci.

Emphysema

Emphysema is a very frequent accompaniment of chronic bronchitis, and it is also seen in some dust diseases of the lungs. It is probable that dust, infections, and noxious fumes are responsible for this condition, but the precise mechanism of causation is not known. In emphysema, the walls of many of the air sacs (alveoli) are destroyed. Examination of an emphysematous lung shows that it is riddled with holes, due to destruction of the normal spongy lung tissue (Figure 10-3).

This means that the surface area of the lung is much reduced. Less oxygen can be absorbed from the air into the blood and the patient may be cyanosed, and less carbon dioxide can be 'blown off'. The accumulation of carbon dioxide in the body gives rise to a respiratory acidosis (see Chapter 1). A patient with emphysema is therefore short of breath, especially on exertion, and this shortness of breath is often so severe as to make him a respiratory cripple.

The extensive destruction of lung tissue means also that many small blood vessels are destroyed, and the amount of blood that can pass through the lungs is much reduced, and this, as previously mentioned, is a cause of chronic venous congestion.

In an attempt to maintain an adequate flow through the lung, the myocardium of the right ventricle may become much thicker. This cardiac compensation in response to lung damage is called *Cor Pulmonale*. The compensation may suffice for some years, but most emphysema patients eventually die of congestive cardiac failure.

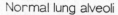

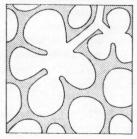 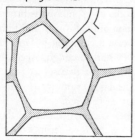

In emphysema, walls of many alveoli destroyed, surface area for gas exchange much reduced and number of capillary blood vessels much reduced

FIG. 10-3 Emphysema

Bronchial Asthma

In this distressing condition, the patient has difficulty in breathing, and it often appears to be more difficult to breathe out than to breathe in. The patients wheeze and are very breathless.

Some cases are due to hypersensitivity to some inhaled substance such as pollen, some are associated with emotional stress, some are due to heredity, some are due to a mixture of all of these factors, and some are not apparently due to any of them. How these factors work is not known, but they all affect the smaller bronchi, which become plugged by a particularly thick and tough mucus, and also the muscle in the wall of these smaller bronchi contracts and this produces further blockage.

In a few severe cases, the condition may develop and persist despite all treatment. This is called *Status Asthmaticus*, and some of these patients die of congestive cardiac failure.

Pneumoconiosis

The long-continued exposure to certain dusts may cause a chronic inflammation and fibrosis known as pneumoconiosis (*konis* = dust). The dangerous element in most kinds of dust is silica, which is present in many kinds of rock. Fine particles of it are produced in most kinds of mining, and in metal grinding and sand-blasting. Most of the particles inhaled are trapped in the slimy mucus lining the airways and they are coughed out, but a few of the smallest particles may reach the alveoli. These are ingested by the alveolar phagocytic cells, and some of them are carried to the lymph nodes at the root of the lung. But the cells are not capable of disposing of the particles, and the particles very slowly dissolve and give off silicic acid which is an irritant. This stimulates the formation of tiny balls of fibrous tissue, and with prolonged irritation these slowly enlarge until they form silicotic nodules of fibrous tissue in the lungs and lymph nodes. The silicic acid is probably also responsible for the destruction of many of the very delicate alveolar walls that make up the lung tissue. The pneumoconioses are therefore characterised by the formation of numerous nodules of fibrous tissue in the lungs, together with destruction of very many of the walls of the alveoli. The condition is progressive as the irritant action of the particles continues for many years, and eventually much of the lung tissue is destroyed. Patients with pneumoconiosis are particularly liable to develop pulmonary tuberculosis as a complication.

In Great Britain, Coal Miner's Pneumoconiosis is the most commonly seen of the dust diseases, and it leads to much disability, though much can be done to prevent it by the use of masks, ventilation and water sprays to keep the dust down in the mines. The lungs of an affected coal miner show extensive tissue destruction and numerous fibrous nodules, and also very marked blackening due to the carbon particles inhaled from the coal. Blackening of the lungs is called *anthracosis*, and it is seen in the lungs of every town dweller, due to the inhalation of soot particles, but fortunately these carbon soot particles do relatively little damage to the lungs and so anthracosis is really a description rather than a disease.

Silica particles are also produced in metal grinding and sand-blasting and they cause a very similar form of pneumoconiosis, the only difference being that as no carbon is inhaled, there is no accompanying anthracosis.

Asbestos is used as insulation and in brake linings. It is composed of fine rod-shaped particles of silica, and it is particularly liable to cause dust disease. The rod-shaped particles can be seen down the microscope and are called asbestos bodies. Asbestosis is bad enough, but the complications are still worse, as quite apart from an increased liability to pulmonary tuberculosis, there is also a marked tendency for carcinoma of the bronchus to develop, and also for a very rare tumour to develop in the pleura called a *mesothelioma*.

Inhalation of the dust from cotton and from sugar cane may cause other lung diseases, called *byssinosis* and *bagassosis* respectively.

Tumours of the Upper Respiratory Tract

Apart from polyps in the nose, which are nearly always of inflammatory origin, tumours of the upper respiratory tract are fortunately uncommon. The larynx and vocal cords are most frequently affected. Fibrotic nodules called 'Singer's nodes' are common and they are not strictly tumours. True tumours of the vocal cords do also occur, some of which are benign and some are malignant.

Carcinoma of the Bronchus (Bronchogenic Carcinoma)

Carcinoma of the bronchus is the commonest of all tumours in men. It arises in the epithelium that lines the bronchus and not in the lung itself.

By far the most important single factor in causing it is cigarette smoking, though presumably there must be other factors as some heavy smokers do not develop cancer, and a few non-smokers do. Town dwellers are more at risk than country dwellers, and perhaps this is due to motor car exhaust fumes, but this factor is much less important than cigarette smoking. Despite the efforts of many researchers we still do not know what it is in cigarette smoke that causes cancer. But cigarette smoke certainly does. A person who regularly smokes twenty or more cigarettes a day has a risk of developing cancer that is more than forty times that of a non-smoker. Pipe smokers are also at risk but the risk is only about a fifth of that of cigarette smokers. In some cases, other factors such as asbestosis or radioactivity may be important.

A patient with carcinoma of the bronchus may have a cough, blood in the sputum (haemoptysis), or pain due to involvement of the pleura. The tumour often blocks one of the large bronchi, and the lung tissue beyond it often becomes airless and it collapses. It is usually also infected, as mucus and bacteria can no longer be removed. Tumour may therefore be suspected in any case of pneumonia that does not respond to treatment within two weeks or so.

X-rays of the chest are used in the investigation, and specimens of sputum or of pleural fluid may be examined microscopically to detect tumour cells. Specimens obtained by bronchoscopy, by needle biopsy of the lung or by removal of a scalene lymph node from just behind the clavicle may also be submitted to microscopic examination to detect the presence of tumour tissue. The terms squamous cell carcinoma, undifferentiated carcinoma, oat-cell carcinoma or adenocarcinoma are used by the pathologist to indicate the various different patterns of tumour growth that may be seen down the microscope.

One of the chief features of bronchial carcinoma is its tendency to metastasise, and secondary tumour deposits may develop even while the original tumour is still quite small. The tumour cells may be carried in lymphatic channels to the lymph nodes in the chest, or they may be carried in the bloodstream to distant sites such as the liver, brain, kidney, bones or adrenal glands. It is for this reason that all patients suspected of having a tumour in the brain are given a chest X-ray, to detect any possible primary source for a secondary tumour deposit in the brain. The tendency for metastases to occur early makes the outlook very poor in this condition, and the number of patients who survive five years or more is less than 3 per cent, and this applies whether or not surgical or radiotherapy or other treatment has been given.

Not all tumours of the bronchi are malignant, as benign tumours do sometimes develop, but they are much less common. Benign tumours give rise to many of the changes seen with malignant tumours, but they do not metastasise, and for this reason surgery is usually effective in these cases.

Bronchiectasis

Bronchiectasis is dilatation of one or more bronchi, rather like an aneurysm, and like an aneurysm it may be due to weakening of the wall. In bronchiectasis, the weakness is probably the result of infection of the wall of the bronchus, and the bulging outwards is probably due to the pressure changes which occur during coughing. Bronchiectasis may follow whooping cough or measles, or it may be a complication of cystic fibrosis.

The result is a stagnant pool of mucus and bacteria which collects in the cavity in the wall of the bronchus, and may spread and give rise to other infections in the lung, or to abscesses in the brain or elsewhere, due to dissemination of the bacteria in the bloodstream.

Pneumothorax
Pneumothorax is air between the lungs and ribs, in the pleural sac. The air usually comes from a small hole in the lung surface, from a rupture of a bulla in emphysema, or due to puncture of the lung by the sharp end of a broken rib. The air in the pleural space presses on the adjacent lung, and part or the whole of one lung collapses and is airless.

Hydrothorax
Fluid in the pleural sacs may have a similar effect. The fluid may collect due to inflammation and be formed as an inflammatory exudate, or it may form as a part of generalised oedema, or it may be pus in empyema, or it may be due to tumour involving the lung surface, and it is then called a malignant pleural effusion.

Pulmonary Embolism and Pulmonary Oedema
These important conditions are described in Chapter 4.

11 *DISEASES OF THE ALIMENTARY TRACT*

THE MOUTH
The Teeth
Caries
Periodontitis

Cancer in the Mouth

THE OESOPHAGUS
Atresia of the Oesophagus

Oesophageal Reflux

Cancer of the Oesophagus

Oesophageal Varices

THE STOMACH
Acute Gastritis

Chronic Gastritis

Peptic Ulcer
Chronic Peptic Ulcer

Cancer of the Stomach

THE INTESTINES
Meckel's Diverticulum

Malabsorption

Infections of the Intestines

Ulcerative Colitis

Acute Intestinal Obstruction

Chronic Intestinal Obstruction

Crohn's Disease (Regional Enteritis)

Appendicitis

Tumours of the Intestines

Diverticulosis and Diverticulitis

Peritonitis: 'The Acute Abdomen'

Ascites

THE MOUTH
The Teeth
A tooth consists of a central stalk of soft tissue called the pulp which contains blood vessels, lymphatic channels and nerves. Around and over the top of this is a cylinder of dentine which is calcified and perforated by numerous minute channels. The part of the dentine which projects above the tooth socket in the jaw is covered with a crown of very hard, somewhat brittle, calcified material called enamel, the hardest material in the whole body. Around the lower part of the dentine there is a layer of cement which contains many fibres to anchor the teeth into the socket of the jaw. The diseases of the teeth which concern us all are caries and periodontitis.

CARIES
Caries means decay, and in the teeth this decay is due to the erosive action of acids on the calcific material of the enamel. Children are the main victims. The acids are produced by the action on food particles of the bacteria which we all carry in our mouths. Food debris may lodge in the crevices between the teeth or in any crack or hollow on the tooth, and the acids accumulate here in sufficient concentration to dissolve away the enamel. Bacteria cannot be removed permanently from our mouths, and so the prevention of dental caries means vigorous up-and-down brushing and reducing sweets. Sweets are both sugary and sticky, and they are particularly liable to produce enough acid to damage the teeth. It seems that biscuits are less harmful to children's teeth than the usual kindly-intentioned offering of 'sweeties'. The dental enamel is much less readily attacked by acids if it contains a small amount of fluorine. To provide the trace of fluorine that is needed, many dentists advocate putting fluorine in drinking water and toothpaste.

The gradual pitting of the enamel may eventually reach the dentine which is less resistant, and this may be eroded to form a cavity, and then bacteria may reach the pulp and set up an acute inflammation of the pulp, which is painful. The process may continue further, and extend down through the pulp to form an abscess beneath and around the root, a root abscess (Figure 11-1).

PERIODONTITIS
The periodontium is the tissue surrounding the root of a tooth, between the root and the tooth socket in the jaw. Periodontitis is an inflammation of this tissue leading to atrophy and eventually to loss of the tooth. The process is seen to some extent in most adults. It starts in the shallow groove around each tooth called the *gingival sulcus*, between the tooth and the surrounding gum. Food debris is difficult to remove from this site, and it may form a persistent film or scale which may become calcified. There is chronic irritation of the gum margin which may, from time to time, become inflamed (gingivitis). For some reason, the gum margin does not usually react by producing granulation tissue, but shrinks away and exposes

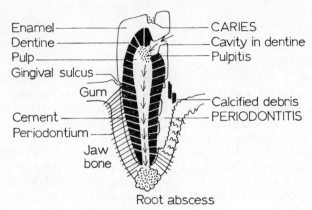

Enamel —————— CARIES
Dentine —————— Cavity in dentine
Pulp —————— Pulpitis
Gingival sulcus
Gum
                                          Calcified debris
Cement —————— PERIODONTITIS
Periodontium
Jaw
bone

Root abscess

FIG. 11-1 Diagram of a tooth, showing the normal structure on the left, and showing the sites of dental caries, root abscess and periodontitis

more and more of the root of the tooth. The process may continue until the periodontium is entirely eroded away, the soft tissue pulp gives way, and the tooth falls out.

Cancer in the Mouth

Cancer is not common in any part of the mouth, but it certainly occurs. In the lips, it is nearly always the lower lip that is affected, and the patients are usually middle-aged or elderly men. The typical story is of an ulcer or whitish, hard patch (leucoplakia) on the lip which is present for years. Eventually the patient complains, and a wedge-shaped piece of lip is surgically removed and microscopic examination shows that cancer is present. The cancer is nearly always indolent and surgical resection is nearly always curative.

Cancer of the tongue usually appears as a lump at the side of the tongue, and it may ulcerate. Cancer of the tongue tends to spread to the lymph nodes in the neck.

Tumours can develop in the salivary glands, especially the parotid salivary gland just in front of the ear. They are mostly *pleomorphic adenomas* (or mixed parotid tumours). These names derive from their microscopic appearances, which need not concern us here. These tumours do not give rise to distant metastases, but they do sometimes recur after surgical excision and this may be because the surgeon has had difficulty in removing all of the tumour without damaging the facial nerve which crosses the region.

Other swellings may develop in the mouth area, most of which are not tumours, but all of which require investigation if they persist for more than a short while.

THE OESOPHAGUS

Swallowing is the only function of the oesophagus and diseases of the oesophagus may cause *dysphagia*, which means difficulty in swallowing. However, not all cases of dysphagia are due to disease of the oesophagus, as the condition is sometimes due to psychological disturbances.

Atresia of the Oesophagus

In this uncommon congenital abnormality, the oesophagus is in the form of a blind pouch, instead of forming a passage to the stomach. At the infant's first feed, the milk cannot enter the stomach, and some of it may spill into the bronchi. The child coughs, turns blue and may very likely develop an aspiration broncho-pneumonia.

Oesophageal Reflux

If you pinch a piece of rubber tubing between finger and thumb, you make a pinch-cock valve that you can open or close at will. The muscle fibres of the diaphragm form a pinch-cock valve around the lower end of the oesophagus. Sometimes this valve action is less than perfect and gastric juice escapes up into the oesophagus—a condition called oesophageal reflux. This is liable to occur when the patient is lying down in bed, and particularly if the pressure in the abdomen is higher than normal, due to obesity, or tight corsets or pregnancy. The irritant gastric acid and pepsin in the oesophagus may cause painful heartburn, or ulceration and inflammation of the epithelial lining of the oesophagus (*reflux oesophagitis*), and this in turn may lead to the formation of a fibrous scar, with subsequent narrowing of the lower end of the oesophagus (*oesophageal stricture*).

Hiatus hernia is a rather ill-defined condition in which the stomach lining is reputed to be drawn up into the diaphragm past the pinch-cock valve, and this may sometimes be the cause or sometimes the result of oesophageal reflux.

Cancer of the Oesophagus

Cancer of the oesophagus arises most commonly at the lower end, though it may occur anywhere. It occurs mainly in middle-aged men and, unfortunately, it seldom causes much dysphagia until it has begun to spread locally into the nearby structures in the chest, making surgery difficult, if not impossible, and it is thus usually eventually fatal.

Oesophageal Varices

Oesophageal varices are dilated, tortuous veins in the wall of the lower end of the oesophagus. They are covered only by the thin lining of the oesophagus which provides them with little protection, and any slight injury from foodstuffs, or the surgeon's oesophagoscope, may precipitate a massive haemorrhage and the vomiting of litres of blood.

As in varicose veins of the legs, oesophageal varices are due to a poor venous circulation. In this case they are due to hypertension in the portal system of veins, the portal hypertension in turn being caused by cirrhosis of the liver.

THE STOMACH
Acute Gastritis

A transient, acute inflammation of the stomach lining may be due to exposure to any of a variety of insults, such as aspirins, alcohol, caffeine, digitalis or corrosive substances. The inflammation is usually transient as the mucosal lining cells of the stomach are normally replaced every 36 hours or so, and this rapid turnover allows any superficial damage to be speedily repaired when the causative agent is removed.

Chronic Gastritis

The term 'chronic gastritis' embraces a hotchpotch of microscopic changes which may be seen in biopsy specimens obtained during gastroscopy. Sometimes the condition is associated with vague complaints of fullness or nausea, but often there are no gastric symptoms.

The changes seen down the microscope include accumulations of inflammatory cells or atrophy of some of the glandular tissue. A severe atrophic gastritis is often, but not always, seen in pernicious anaemia, and the atrophy probably accounts for the absence of intrinsic factor and the complete absence of acid secretion (achlorhydria) which are constant features of pernicious anaemia (Chapter 9).

Peptic Ulcer

Acute ulceration of the superficial lining of the stomach probably occurs fairly commonly but the true incidence is unknown as such lesions heal very rapidly.

CHRONIC PEPTIC ULCER

Chronic peptic ulcers are among the commonest of all human afflictions. Though seldom fatal, they cause much pain and discomfort. It has been estimated that 10 per cent of the population at one time or another suffer from peptic ulcers, men more commonly than women.

The peptic juice contains hydrochloric acid and the powerful digestive enzyme pepsin. Peptic ulcers occur in those parts of the lining of the alimentary tract which are exposed to the action of the peptic juice.

The first part of the *duodenum* is the commonest site, and ulcers here are four or five times commoner than those in the stomach. In the *stomach*, peptic ulcers may develop in the funnel-shaped area called the pyloric antrum, which leads to the pylorus and duodenum. The ulcers are found usually between 5 and 10 cm from the pylorus, most commonly along the upper border (lesser curvature) of the stomach.

Occasionally, peptic ulcers occur at the lower end of the *oesophagus*, if there is oesophageal reflux; in the lining of a *Meckel's diverticulum*; or sometimes, after a gastroenterostomy, in the first part of the jejunum where an opening into it is formed directly from the stomach (*stomal ulcer*).

In chronic peptic ulceration, there is ulceration right through the lining of the bowel and into the muscle layer. The ulcer takes the form of a crater up to 5 cm diameter. It has sharply punched-out edges, with a smooth, clean floor due to peptic digestion of any exudate. The floor of an ulcer may consist of the outer part of the stomach wall which is usually very considerably thickened by a large amount of fibrosis. Fibrous tissue tends to contract after it has formed, and in the wall of the stomach this produces folds in the stomach lining which radiate from the ulcer and provide a valuable clue to the location of the ulcer for the surgeon, the radiologist and the pathologist.

Sometimes the ulcers extend right through the wall of the stomach, and the floor of the ulcer is formed of fibrous tissue in the adjacent organs, such as pancreas, liver or bile ducts.

The fibrosis which occurs at the base of an ulcer may produce a severe constriction, especially in the stomach, and it may result in a partial obstruction known as *pyloric stenosis.*

Perforation is a very serious complication of peptic ulcer, in which a hole develops right through the wall of the stomach or duodenum through which bacteria and peptic juice may pour into the peritoneal cavity, causing peritonitis.

Haemorrhage is the other important complication. If the haemorrhage is slight, it may appear like coffee grounds in any vomited material. Sometimes the blood is not vomited but appears as a black colour in the faeces (*melaena*). If the haemorrhage is due to the erosion of an artery, there may be a massive vomiting of fresh blood known as *haematemesis.*

PEPTIC ULCER—CAUSATION

The immediate cause of a peptic ulcer is the digestive action of the peptic juice. People with high levels of acid in the gastric juice are more liable to ulcers than normal people. Nervous stress is known to raise the level of acid production. Patients with little or no peptic juice, due to removal or atrophy of the stomach, do not get ulcers and ulcers seldom develop in the second part of the duodenum as in this region the acid in the peptic juice is neutralised by the bile and the pancreatic secretions.

Normally, the secretion of slimy mucus affords protection from the effects of the peptic juice, and in any case of superficial erosion, the lining cells rapidly multiply to heal the damage. There is thus normally a balance between the destructive effect of the juices and these two protective mechanisms. Presumably, in peptic ulceration some local change in the lining occurs which decreases both mucus production and the healing capacity, and upsets the balance. There have been many theories as to the basis of this change, ranging from local ischaemia to virus infection, but it remains a mystery.

Until this mystery is solved, the treatment of peptic ulcer can only be aimed at decreasing the amount of acid present, by giving alkali tablets to neutralise it, by removing the acid-forming part of the stomach, or by cutting the vagus nerves which stimulate acid secretion.

Cancer of the Stomach

Cancer of the stomach is almost as common as cancer of the bronchus, and in some countries it is the most common malignant tumour.

The tumours develop in the glands in the lining of the stomach, and consist of a mass of poorly-formed gland-like structures (*adenocarcinoma*). The tumours grow rapidly, both within the stomach and out through the wall of the stomach. Inside the stomach, the centre of the tumour often ulcerates, and this produces a ring of tumour tissue surrounding an ulcer crater. Outside the stomach, there is rapid spread to the lymph nodes and to the liver. Unfortunately, the patient seldom experiences much discomfort or vomiting until the tumour has spread widely, and for this reason the outlook is very poor and few patients survive a year from the time of diagnosis.

With gastric carcinoma, the detection of blood in the faeces may be the first indication that something is wrong. The other investigations required usually include X-ray examination after ingesting a barium solution to outline the tumour; microscopic examination of the cells in the gastric juice; gastroscopy measurement of the amount of acid in the gastric juice, as it is often low in gastric carcinoma (*hypochlorhydria*).

The stomach lining is exposed to all the food and noxious agents we eat and it may be that one or more of these agents is responsible for the development of tumours. The highest incidence of gastric carcinoma occurs in countries like Finland, Iceland, Chile and Japan, in all of which a lot of fish is eaten. But investigation of fish and the substances they contain has so far proved entirely negative, and we are still almost entirely ignorant of the causes of carcinoma of the stomach.

THE INTESTINES
Meckel's Diverticulum
Meckel's diverticulum is a congenital abnormality which takes the form of a pouch in the wall of the small intestine, usually near the lower end. Sometimes the cells lining the diverticulum include acid-secreting gland cells, as in the stomach, and occasionally these cells may be the cause of a peptic ulcer, but much more frequently the diverticulum causes no trouble and is found incidentally during abdominal operations.

Malabsorption
The two main functions of the intestines are the digestion of the food into small molecules and the absorption of these molecules. Malabsorption may be due to failure of either of these processes. Poor absorption from the intestines is rather like starvation. It causes a shortage of essential nutriments, especially of protein and the fat-soluble vitamins A, D and K. It is commonest in children. Normally there are millions of very small folds (villi) in the lining of the intestine for the absorption of digested food, but in many of these children the villi are small or absent. The affected children are small for their age, fail to thrive, do not put on weight, suffer more infections than usual and they often have persistent diarrhoea with fatty acid stools.

In adults, and also sometimes in children, malabsorption may be due principally to poor digestion of the food due to disease in the pancreas or gall-bladder or elsewhere. A deficiency of the digestive enzymes in the pancreatic juice may result from pancreatic disease, such as fibrocystic disease or it may be due to blockage of the pancreatic ducts by a gall-stone.

Infections of the Intestines
In western countries, where reasonable sanitation exists, it is difficult to appreciate that, in other parts of the world, enormous numbers of deaths are caused by intestinal infections, and that often the victims are infants and young children.

The infections responsible are the enteric fevers including typhoid, food poisoning, gastro-enteritis, dysentery due to either bacteria or amoebae, and cholera.

Typhoid fever is due to the organism *Salmonella typhi*, which is carried in water and occasionally in meat. If ingested, the organism passes through the lining of the gut into the adjacent lymphoid tissue where it multiplies. The lining of the gut overlying the lymphoid tissue may ulcerate. The organism enters the bloodstream and all the lymph nodes in the body become infected. Continued multiplication of the organism may lead to severe toxaemia and death from shock due to the release of bacterial toxins. Thus, typhoid fever commences as an infection of the gut, but rapidly spreads to affect the lymphoid tissue and then the whole body.

The other enteric fevers are due to other varieties of Salmonella organisms such as Paratyphoid B. The disease process is very similar to typhoid, but usually less severe, and seldom causes death.

Food poisoning may be caused by other varieties of Salmonella bacteria, of which *Salmonella typhi-murium* is the commonest in Great Britain. These organisms infect the lining of the intestines and the lymph nodes and they cause severe diarrhoea. Food poisoning due to *Clostridium welchii*, the organism which in other circumstances can cause Gas Gangrene, is similar to food poisoning due to Salmonellae. Staphylococcal food poisoning is due not so much to ingested bacteria as to ingested toxins. Staphylococci are very liable to multiply and produce toxins in any infected food, especially if the food is kept warm and moist for any period of time. The victim thus ingests ready-made toxins, which cause inflammation of the lining of the stomach, and vomiting within an hour or so of eating of the food.

Gastro-enteritis is a superficial inflammation of the lining of the stomach and intestines. It may be due to any of a variety of bacterial organisms or some viruses. Vomiting may be the principal feature if the stomach is involved, or diarrhoea and dehydration if the intestines are affected. Recovery occurs after a few days of misery.

Dysentery means diarrhoea with blood, pus and mucus in the faeces, and usually with pain on defaecation and shock. Bacillary dysentery is caused by a group of bacteria called *Shigella*, which is conveyed on food contaminated by the hands of an infected person. The organism has a direct action on the lining of the intestine, which is stripped off in patches. The shock is mostly due to dehydration but may, in part, be due to the effect of an endotoxin entering the bloodstream and causing dilatation of the arterioles. Death is uncommon in adults.

Amoebic dysentery occurs in tropical countries and sometimes in mental hospitals. It is due to infection by the organism *Entamoeba histolytica*. The features are similar to those of bacillary dysentery, except that there is little or no pus in the faeces. Occasionally the organisms spread to the liver and give rise to an *amoebic abscess* there.

Cholera is endemic in parts of the Far East, and the great epidemics of cholera that from time to time sweep across Asia as far as Turkey originate in the Far East. The *Vibrio cholera* is a water-borne organism that gives rise to severe inflammation of the lining of the intestines if ingested, with a very rapid loss of fluid into the bowel, and with loss of curls of the lining epithelium which gives the faeces the appearance of 'rice water'. The dehydration due to the loss of fluid in the faeces may be very severe, and it is possible for a child to lose a quarter of its body weight in 24 hours, and to be profoundly and sometimes fatally shocked. Fluid loss leading to dehydration is one of the principal pathological processes in all the intestinal infections mentioned and it may become severe before other pathological changes, due to bacterial invasion, have time to appear.

Ulcerative Colitis

This distressing condition is mentioned here as some of its features are similar to those of intestinal infections but there are two major differences. One is that the cause of ulcerative colitis is unknown, and the other is that the disease tends to last for many years with acute flare-ups from time to time. The other features resemble those of the intestinal infections. There is diarrhoea, with mucus, pus and blood in the faeces and there may be dehydration. The disease affects mainly the large intestine, which may show very extensive necrosis and ulceration of the lining. Between each attack there may be some regeneration of the lining of the colon with the formation of numerous little polyps.

Acute Intestinal Obstruction

In acute intestinal obstruction, the normal peristaltic waves of contraction in the wall of the intestine above the blockage become more vigorous in an attempt to force the intestinal contents along. There is a build-up of pressure, and only a moderate increase of pressure is required to cause the veins in the wall of the intestine to collapse, with the result that no blood can leave the affected bowel. It becomes oedematous and congested with blood until, after an hour or so, it is so congested that no more blood can come along the arteries and the arterial supply stops. The cells in the bowel wall start to die and it is only a matter of time then before bacteria from the intestine escape into the peritoneal cavity and cause peritonitis. A patient with acute intestinal obstruction has an urgent need of surgical help.

Acute intestinal obstruction affects the small intestine much more commonly than the large intestine. The patient suffers acute colicky pain, shock and collapse and there is often complete constipation and vomiting.

The affected bowel is distended by an accumulation within it of digestive juice, oedema fluid and blood, and the fluid loss may be so great as to cause dehydration and shock. The quantity of fluid accumulating within the intestine may be visible on X-rays and this is what is meant by the term 'fluid levels on X-ray'. The wall of the bowel is congested so as to be thickened and it looks purple from the quantity of stagnant blood in it. At operation, after relieving the cause of the obstruction, the surgeon may attempt to restore the blood flow by applying warm towels to the affected bowel. If the colour of the bowel does not revert to normal within a few minutes, the affected portion must be cut out and the two normal ends joined together.

Acute intestinal obstruction may occur if the nerve cells in the wall of the intestine, which control the normal waves of peristaltic contraction, are damaged (*paralytic ileus*) by excessive handling at operation or by peritonitis. Thrombosis of the arterial blood supply to the intestine such as *mesenteric artery thrombosis* may have a similar effect. However, the commonest causes of acute intestinal obstruction are mechanical ones, such as peritoneal adhesions, hernias, intussusception and volvulus (Figure 11-2).

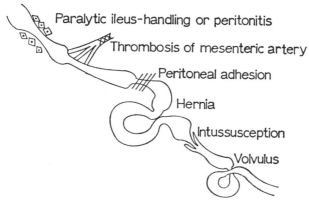

FIG. 11-2 Diagrammatic representation of the common causes of acute intestinal obstruction

Peritoneal adhesions are bands of fibrous tissue which develop following inflammation and fibrin exudation. They may be due to healing and repair after abdominal operations or they may follow some previous incident of inflammation such as acute appendicitis.

A *hernia* is a protrusion of a loop of bowel through an opening or weak point in the wall of the abdominal cavity. The common site for such a protrusion is in the groin (inguinal and femoral hernias). Such a protrusion may cause discomfort. It only becomes serious if part of the bowel becomes trapped by the tissues at the neck of the hernia pouch (strangulation). The affected portion of bowel may be grooved at each end by the neck of the hernia pouch, and the pressure change involved may initiate the dramatic changes of acute intestinal obstruction.

Intussusception is a curious cause of acute intestinal obstruction which occurs in children. The usual site is at, or near, the junction of the small and large intestines. For some reason, a segment of small bowel may be dragged by peristaltic contractions into the first part of the large bowel. Intussusception is thus a telescoping of one part of the bowel into another. Again the pressure changes interfere with the venous drainage of the bowel, and the other changes of acute obstruction follow.

A *volvulus* is a twist, and sometimes a segment of the bowel may become twisted up on itself. Why this should happen is not known but the result, once again, is acute intestinal obstruction.

Chronic Intestinal Obstruction

In contrast to acute obstruction, chronic intestinal obstruction occurs most commonly in the large intestine. The commonest cause is a tumour developing in the wall of the large bowel. The tumour produces a partial obstruction to the flow of intestinal contents and this often produces a pattern of alternating constipation and diarrhoea. The bowel upstream from the obstruction may be hugely distended by hard faecal material (*megacolon*). Megacolon is also present in a form of chronic intestinal obstruction known as *Hirschsprung's disease*, which occurs in infants and young children. It is due to a congenital absence of the nerves which produce peristaltic contractions in the wall of the rectum. If untreated, the obstruction may become more complete and the patient may suffer persistent vomiting, dehydration and loss of potassium.

Crohn's Disease (Regional Enteritis)

Crohn's disease is one of the exceptions to the general rule that chronic intestinal obstruction occurs mainly in the large bowel. In this condition it is mainly the small bowel which is affected, especially the last metre or so of the small bowel. The changes seen are those of chronic inflammation, with the formation of numerous granulomas and much fibrous tissue in the wall of the small intestine, nearly always associated with some degree of ulceration of the lining. The cause of the condition remains a mystery. A feature of the disease is that some patches of the small intestine are affected and other areas show no change. Each of the affected patches becomes thick-walled and rigid, like a length of hose-pipe, with intervening areas of normal, delicate and flexible bowel wall. The wall becomes so rigid that the peristaltic waves of muscular contraction cannot pass along, and the patients suffer rather vague abdominal pain due to obstruction, with bouts of diarrhoea and often some blood in the faeces. The disease runs a prolonged course, sometimes with acute exacerbations. Occasionally there is malabsorption, and sometimes cracks and fissures develop and fistulae may form between one loop of the bowel and another.

Appendicitis

As far as is known, the appendix serves no useful function whatsoever, but it is of considerable medical importance on account of the frequency of acute appendicitis and the fact that peritonitis may follow. The appendix is a little blind tube that opens out of the junction of the small and large intestines. Occasionally the tube may become obstructed by a grape pip, a lead shot or a hardened pellet of faecal material, but much more commonly obstruction is due to inflammation in the neck of the tube. The inflamed tissue swells and blocks the tube and the bacteria beyond the blockage multiply unhindered and pus accumulates in the tube. The wall of the appendix may be eroded by the effect of bacterial toxins or of pressure on the venous drainage, just as in any other form of acute intestinal obstruction. The pressure may be considerable as, unlike the rest of the alimentary tract, an obstructed appendix is closed at both ends. The inner, and then the outer layers of the wall of the appendix become necrotic. If untreated, the appendix is very liable to burst, scattering bacteria and faecal material into the peritoneal cavity.

In most hospitals, appendectomy for acute appendicitis is the commonest of all surgical operations. Some cases of acute appendicitis would probably heal by themselves without causing peritonitis if allowed to do so, but unfortunately no one can tell which patients are going to heal and which to develop peritonitis. It is curious that the disease is uncommon in under-developed countries and that it was almost unheard of in this country until one hundred years ago.

Tumours of the Intestines

Tumours of the small intestine are uncommon. In the alimentary tract, the common sites for tumours are the stomach and large bowel, with the oesophagus running a poor third. Carcinomas in either of these sites are only a little less common than the commonest of all malignant tumours, carcinoma of the bronchus. In the large intestine, the rectum and the sigmoid colon are the most frequent site of tumour development. A carcinoma of the large intestine arises in the lining of the bowel and slowly enlarges. The developing tumour gradually produces narrowing of the bowel and chronic intestinal obstruction occurs. The tumour may bleed and there may be blood in the faeces which can be tested. The tumours can often be seen directly as they are often within range of the sigmoidoscope. The tumours infiltrate the wall of the bowel and into the lymph nodes, but in contrast to carcinoma of the stomach, this happens fairly slowly and there is a moderately good chance of a complete cure by surgery if the diagnosis can be made early enough. An alteration in bowel habit is often the earliest change.

Many tumours of the large bowel are benign and not invasive. They take the form of polyps and adenomas arising in the mucosal lining of the bowel, and they may bleed or cause partial obstruction.

Multiple polyposis coli has been mentioned earlier as an example of one of the few hereditary conditions that give rise to cancer, but this only accounts for a very few cases of carcinoma of the large bowel.

Diverticulosis and Diverticulitis

There is good evidence to suggest that diverticulosis is due to increased pressure in the large bowel, due to the increased peristaltic waves of contraction that occur in constipation. It is thought that the pressure forces the delicate lining of the bowel out through any weak places in the muscle layer to form small pouches, each about the size of a pea (*diverticulosis*).

Often such diverticulae cause no trouble, but sometimes they become inflamed (*diverticulitis*). This may be painful, rather like acute appendicitis, but sometimes there is little discomfort for the patient, and the diverticulum becomes surrounded by a mass of fibrous tissue. This lump of fibrous tissue may be mistaken for a carcinoma until a microscopic examination of the tissue is made.

Peritonitis: 'The Acute Abdomen'

The peritoneum is a thin membrane which has many folds in it and covers the outer surfaces of the intestines and lines the abdominal cavity. Bacteria may enter this cavity and initiate widespread inflammation of the intestines if any part of the intestines are perforated. The commonest cause of this is the rupture of an acutely inflamed appendix. Less commonly, an acutely infected gall-bladder or a peptic ulcer may perforate.

Other causes of perforation include Crohn's disease, ulcerative colitis, diverticulitis of the colon or ulcerating carcinomas of the stomach or large intestines, and
any of the forms of acute intestinal obstruction may also lead to perforation due to
gangrene of the bowel wall.

Sometimes the bacteria may be localised to one part of the peritoneum, by the
rapid development of inflammation and fibrinous adhesions between the nearest
adjacent parts of the intestines. The bacteria are thus trapped and an abscess forms,
such as an appendix abscess around a perforated appendix.

In other cases, the bacteria spread throughout the peritoneal cavity. Early
changes include shock, a board-like rigidity of the muscles of the anterior wall of
the abdomen, and the production by bacteria of gas which collects under the
diaphragm and can be seen as a bubble on X-rays. Inflammation occurs on the
peritoneal surface all over the intestines and produces a paralytic ileus, by affecting
the nerve cells which control the peristaltic contraction waves. The effect is an
acute intestinal obstruction in which not one area but the whole length of the
intestine is involved. The consequent fluid loss and dehydration which follow
produce a catastrophic fall in blood pressure.

It should be mentioned that pancreatic juice or blood in the peritoneal cavity
can produce a very similar inflammation. Pancreatic juice, which contains powerful digestive enzymes, may be released into the peritoneal cavity in acute pancreatitis. Blood may escape into the cavity from a tubal pregnancy or, less often,
by rupture of an aneurysm of the aorta.

In all these conditions, except acute pancreatitis, the only possible treatment is
restoration of the blood pressure followed by surgery. In acute pancreatitis, surgery
is seldom desirable.

Ascites

Ascites is the name used for a collection of fluid in the peritoneal cavity. This may
occur as part of a generalised oedema affecting the whole body, in which case
oedema may be present in the sacrum, ankles, scrotum, pleural and pericardial
cavities as well. Inflammation or tumour involving the peritoneum may also cause
ascites, but the most dramatic examples are those due to obstruction of the portal
venous drainage of the intestines, usually due to cirrhosis of the liver. In these cases,
enormous volumes of fluid may be repeatedly withdrawn from the peritoneal
cavity.

12 DISEASES OF THE LIVER AND GALL-BLADDER

THE LIVER
Liver Cell Damage

Jaundice

Cirrhosis

Other Diseases Affecting the Liver

THE GALL-BLADDER

THE LIVER

The liver is the largest single organ in the body. It acts as a chemical workshop, in which a large number of chemical processes take place, all performed by one kind of cell. The liver cells have been extensively studied by electron microscopy and they are found to contain a variety of microscopic structures in their cytoplasm, which enable them to perform the many different chemical reactions required. The liver has a large reserve capacity, and it is possible for a large number of liver cells to be destroyed before any change in function is seen. If the liver cells are destroyed, the remaining ones can readily multiply to make good the loss.

The liver is provided with a complex network of channels consisting of bile ducts and three kinds of blood vessels. The bile ducts drain away the bile formed by the liver cells and convey it to the gall-bladder and hence eventually to the duodenum. The blood vessels of the liver are the portal vein, the hepatic artery and the hepatic vein. The portal vein is formed by the joining together of the veins from the stomach, the small and large intestines and the spleen. It carries blood to the liver, together with molecules of digested foodstuffs. The other blood supply is the hepatic artery, which is similar to any other artery in the body. It supplies blood to the liver at a much higher pressure than the portal vein. The hepatic vein provides the venous drainage for the blood from both the portal vein and the hepatic artery. Each of these systems has a large number of small branches, so that each individual liver cell is adjacent to a branch from each system. It will be appreciated then that the liver is interlaced with a complex network of channels, arterial, portal, venous and biliary.

Liver Cell Damage

Viruses and various toxic chemicals are the agents that most commonly cause damage to the liver cells. The two viruses principally concerned are those of infectious hepatitis and serum hepatitis (hepatitis A and hepatitis B). They both invade and kill liver cells, and this is followed by an acute inflammation in the liver.

The virus of infectious hepatitis is transmitted by ingestion of infected food or drink. Important preventative measures against this disease include washing of hands, good sanitation, suppression of flies and avoidance of suspect shellfish. Dr Pickles, a Yorkshire family doctor, demonstrated, by careful observation of its spread in an isolated community, that the disease has an incubation period of up to about forty days. Approximately 85 per cent of the individuals affected show little illness. They are asymptomatic carriers. Some may have a 'flu-like' illness. Others develop jaundice, which persists for a few weeks and is nearly always followed by complete recovery.

The virus of serum hepatitis is transmitted in blood or blood products from an infected individual. The quantity of blood required to transmit the virus is very small, and the infection may be transmitted, for instance, in traces of blood on an inadequately sterilised syringe needle if one of the people injected carries the virus.

Blood or plasma used for blood transfusion is another source of infection. It has been estimated that approximately one out of every 800 units of blood used for transfusion contains the virus, acquired from an infected but symptomless and unsuspecting blood donor, who may carry the virus in his blood for a year, or sometimes much longer, following his initial infection. The persons most at risk of developing serum hepatitis are patients who need large quantities of donor blood, such as patients with haemolytic anaemias, or those on dialysis for chronic renal failure. There is a long incubation period of anything from 40 to 120 days, and then liver cell damage shows as jaundice. The disease tends to be more severe than infectious hepatitis and though it generally subsides, it is fatal in a few cases. The infected patients harbour large numbers of the virus in their blood. Nurses and doctors in contact with them run a risk of infection from any accidental skin break or via any slight abrasion. Nurses and doctors who do become infected may suffer a particularly severe form of the disease. It has been suggested that this is because their healthy, antibody-forming and cellular immune mechanisms react more strongly to the infection than do those of severely ill patients, and that it is the violence of the immune response which contributes to the severity of the disease.

Most people who are infected by the serum hepatitis virus have fragments of the virus in their blood. This fragment is called the Australia Antigen (HBsAg). A gel-diffusion test has recently been developed to detect this fragment. It is found in most, but not all, cases of serum hepatitis infection, and it is also present in the blood of some symptomless carriers. It has also been found incidentally in about half of all cases of *polyarteritis nodosa*, but the significance of this finding is not known. The use of this test for the Australia Antigen has made it possible in most cases to detect the virus in donor blood for transfusion, and by this method it is hoped to prevent most cases of infection by transfused blood.

Some toxic chemicals have very similar effects on the liver to those of the hepatitis viruses. The chemicals are absorbed by the intestines and carried to the liver in the portal venous blood. The chemicals may produce extensive liver cell damage, with jaundice and occasionally death, but more often with residual changes in the structure of the liver. Carbon tetrachloride, which is used as a cleaning fluid, chloroform and Yellow Phosphorus are examples of these chemicals. The liver cell damage that is produced results in numerous biochemical changes, the most obvious of which is a raised level of bilirubin in the blood, which is seen as jaundice. When the liver cells are damaged, they release enzymes into the blood and this can be demonstrated by chemical tests to show the increased levels of the enzymes SGOT (serum glutamic oxylate transaminase) and SICD (serum iso-citrate dehydrogenase) in the blood.

Jaundice

Jaundice is the name for the yellow colour of the skin and the whites of the eyes due to an increased level of bilirubin in the blood. It occurs when the amount of bilirubin formed by the breakdown of red blood cells is much increased, or if the capacity of the liver to process and excrete bilirubin is reduced.

The rate of red cell breakdown is sometimes enormously increased in Haemolytic anaemias. Jaundice may occur, but it is seldom severe unless liver damage is also present (due sometimes to haemosiderosis or serum hepatitis following blood transfusion), as the normal liver has a considerable unused extra capacity.

The commonest cause of jaundice is liver cell damage, in which the processing and excretion of bilirubin is impaired, and the common causes of this, as already mentioned, are virus hepatitis or toxic chemicals.

Some of the most severe cases of jaundice are due to obstruction of the bile ducts, common causes of which are gall-stones in the ducts, or carcinoma of the head of the pancreas which surrounds the lower end of the duct. Such obstructions prevent the bile from entering the duodenum. The liver cells continue to secrete bile into the bile ducts, until the pressure in the bile ducts becomes too great and secretion fails. In obstructive jaundice, the level of the enzyme alkaline phosphatase in the blood is usually markedly increased, and as no bile reaches the intestine, the faeces are very pale and putty-coloured and the urine dark.

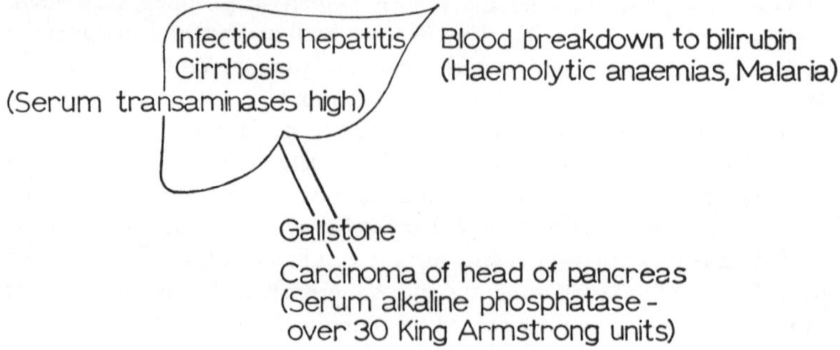

Infectious hepatitis
Cirrhosis
(Serum transaminases high)

Blood breakdown to bilirubin
(Haemolytic anaemias, Malaria)

Gallstone
Carcinoma of head of pancreas
(Serum alkaline phosphatase -
over 30 King Armstrong units)

FIG. 12-1 The causes of jaundice

Cirrhosis

Cirrhosis is an anatomical change in the structure of the liver, which is sometimes associated with impaired liver function. The anatomical change consists of a combination of fibrosis with islands or nodules of regenerated liver cells. This appearance appears to indicate that some severe damage has previously occurred to the liver cells, and that the fibrosis and regeneration are the results of repair. Many patients with cirrhosis do have a history of previous jaundice or of some other indication of previous liver cell damage, but in some cases there is no such history. In such cases one can only presume that these persons have developed cirrhosis due to an insidious and slowly progressive liver cell damage without any acute incident.

The cirrhotic liver is firm or even hard due to the proliferation of fibrous tissue, and it consists entirely of nodules of rather yellow and fatty liver cells. In many cases there is a history of previous viral hepatitis, or of repeated excessive alcohol intake, or of other toxic chemical exposure, or evidence of severe congestive cardiac failure. Some cases are associated with malnutrition, but it was noted that little cirrhosis was seen in the survivors from the concentration camps of World War II. It seems probable that malnutrition by itself does not cause cirrhosis, but that it may render the liver cells less capable of resisting the effects of other agents. Perhaps the form of cirrhosis commonly seen in West Africa is due to a combination of malnutrition and some other factor. The same combination of circumstances may account for the cirrhosis seen in chronic alcoholics, as most alcoholics eat very little although they take in a lot of alcohol.

Cirrhosis may also occur in disturbances of iron metabolism. In haemachromatosis, too much iron is absorbed by the alimentary tract (Chapter 9). In *haemosiderosis*, excessive quantities of iron-containing pigment are produced due to excess red cell breakdown, and this occurs in the haemolytic anaemias if treated by massive transfusions. In both cases, large quantities of iron-containing pigment accumulate in the liver, and in other organs, and liver cell damage may occur.

The anatomical changes of cirrhosis particularly upset the complicated arrangement of blood vessels and bile ducts in the liver. For instance, the high-pressure hepatic arterial blood supply may impinge on the low-pressure portal venous blood supply and the portal blood pressure may be unnaturally raised. This may account for some of the features which are commonly associated with cirrhosis, such as thrombosis of the portal vein, dilatation and enlargement of the spleen, the development of widely dilated veins in the wall of the oesophagus (oesophageal varices), and the seepage of fluid through the walls of the small blood vessels of the intestines into the peritoneal space resulting in large amounts of fluid collecting in the abdomen (ascites).

The anatomical changes of the liver may cause changes in the chemical functions of the liver, and there may be mild jaundice. There may also be mental disturbances or even coma, possibly due to raised levels of ammonia in the blood, due to failure of the liver cells to convert ammonia derived from digested protein materials into urea which can be excreted in the urine. Other changes which almost certainly have a biochemical basis include atrophy of the testes, vascular naevi developing in the skin, purpuric bleeding, perhaps due to failure of the liver to form one of the chemicals concerned in blood coagulation, and anaemia.

Other Diseases Affecting the Liver

Many diseases may affect the liver, but the damage they produce is seldom enough to exceed the reserve capacity of the liver or cause jaundice.

Bacterial infections may reach the liver via the portal bloodstream from the intestines or in the hepatic arterial blood supply, and occasionally abscesses may form in the liver. The organism *Entamoeba histolytica* which causes amoebic dysentery may be carried in the portal blood to the liver and give rise to an amoebic abscess, and tapeworm scolices may occasionally travel by the same route to give rise to hydatid cysts in the liver.

Tumour metastases from carcinomas of the stomach or large intestine are very commonly carried in the portal bloodstream to give rise to secondary tumour deposits in the liver. The liver may also receive tumour metastases from the general circulation via the hepatic artery, and the liver is thus one of the commonest sites for secondary tumour deposits to develop.

Primary tumours of the liver cells are rare in Great Britain. They are, however, common in Mozambique, often in association with cirrhosis, and it has been suggested that this may in some way be due to a chemical substance called *aflatoxin*, which is absorbed from the intestine after eating mouldy peanuts or groundnuts.

THE GALL-BLADDER

The gall-bladder is an ancillary organ to the liver. The bile formed by the liver cells passes down the bile ducts and into the gall-bladder where it is stored, and where some of the water is removed to concentrate the bile. When required, the bile passes from the gall-bladder back into the bile duct and down into the duodenum. Bile assists in the digestion of fat in the food. Without bile, for instance in obstructive jaundice, especially if of long duration, a deficiency of fat-soluble vitamins (A, D and K) may occur.

Two diseases commonly affect the gall-bladder, inflammation (*cholecystitis*) and calculus formation (*cholelithiasis*). They very often occur together. Cholecystitis by itself is due to bacterial infection of the gall-bladder, either from bacteria in the blood or by infection ascending up the bile duct from the duodenum. There is intense inflammation with pus formation. As the infection subsides, water is absorbed from the necrotic debris in the gall-bladder, which solidifies, and often calcification occurs in the debris.

Calculus formation in the gall-bladder is often due to infection, but occasionally is due to other causes such as excess bile production in haemolytic anaemias. Usually, however, inflammation and stone formation occur together. The situation is similar to that in the urinary tract, in which the three factors, infection, stasis and obstruction are so interlinked that when one occurs the other two frequently follow, and between them they often give rise to stone formation. Gall-stones may cause obstruction at the neck of the gall-bladder, with pain and dilatation of the gall-bladder. Or they may pass into the bile ducts and cause colicky pain and obstructive jaundice if they are not passed into the duodenum.

Cancer may develop in the gall-bladder, but this is not common. The gall-bladder is, however, one of the sites in the abdomen where a cancer may become quite large before being suspected by either the patient or his physician. The other sites where this may occur are in the tail of the pancreas and in the caecum.

13 *DISEASES OF THE PANCREAS*

Pancreatitis

Diabetes Mellitus
Causes
The Chemical and Other Effects of Diabetes
Diabetic Coma
Complications of Diabetes

Cystic Fibrosis

Tumours of the Pancreas
Carcinoma
Insulin-secreting Tumours

The pancreas is most conveniently considered as two separate glandular organs. The bulk of the pancreatic glandular tissue is concerned with the manufacture of about two litres per day of alkaline secretion. This pancreatic secretion contains the powerful digestive enzymes, trypsin, lipase and amylase, which are respectively concerned with the digestion of protein, fat and carbohydrate. The secretion passes along the pancreatic ducts and into the duodenum through an opening which is shared with the common bile duct.

Scattered through the pancreas are the Islets of Langerhans. These are small groups of cells, most of which manufacture insulin. This hormone, after secretion into the blood, stimulates the absorption of glucose from the blood into the cells of the body, where the glucose can be utilised to produce energy.

Pancreatitis

Pancreatitis is sometimes an acute and sometimes a chronic condition, but as far as is known, there is no basic difference between the two forms of the disease.

There is little doubt that pancreatitis is a form of auto-digestion which is due to the release within the pancreas itself of its own powerful digestive enzymes. There is, however, considerable debate as to why these enzymes are released in the pancreas and not in the duodenum. It is probable that obstruction of the pancreatic ducts is the main cause. It is postulated that in some cases the smaller pancreatic ducts become obstructed by cellular changes in their walls. In some cases, the obstruction may be due to failure of the opening into the duodenum to open, and in other cases the opening may be blocked by a gall-stone. Certainly gall-stones are present in some cases of pancreatitis. About half of all cases of pancreatitis are associated with alcoholism, but it is not known why this should be.

When acute, pancreatitis presents with a sudden onset of very severe pain, often coming on after a meal or a drink. Sometimes, the pain is somewhat eased if the patient sits up and leans forwards. The digestive enzymes may dissolve and destroy parts of the pancreas, and they may escape into the surrounding tissues. They may dissolve some of the blood vessels in and around the pancreas and cause extensive haemorrhage. The digestive enzymes may also attack the fatty tissue near the pancreas, producing numerous white flecks of partly digested fat in the mesentery. The enzymes may escape into the peritoneal cavity and give rise to an acute peritonitis, and this may be the cause of the shock which is sometimes severe. Digestive enzymes are not normally present in any quantity in the blood, but in pancreatitis they may be found in the blood in large amounts. The most readily measured enzyme is serum amylase, which may be raised to very high levels in acute pancreatitis.

When the disease takes a chronic form, the principal troubles are the attacks of severe abdominal pain. The changes described in acute pancreatitis also occur in chronic pancreatitis, but are less severe and less widespread.

Diabetes Mellitus

Diabetes is a common and complex disease. There are about a quarter of a million known diabetics in Britain. The basic abnormality in diabetes is that the level of glucose sugar in the blood is much higher than normal, while inside the cells it is very low. Diabetes is a complex disease as it has four or more different possible causes, and numerous complications, most of which are the result of changes in the arteries and small blood vessels.

CAUSES

In diabetes, the cells are less capable than normal of taking in sugar from the blood. In some cases this is due to a deficient production of insulin by the pancreas, but in many cases the production of insulin is normal or even higher than normal, and in these cases some other explanation than insulin deficiency must be sought.

Some diabetics may require 500 or even 1000 units of insulin every day to control the blood sugar level. This is far more than the pancreas normally produces. This increased insulin requirement may be due to the presence of insulin antagonists. These are other hormones which have effects directly or indirectly opposite to that of insulin, i.e. they tend to raise the blood sugar. For instance, growth hormone produced by the pituitary gland can contribute to diabetes by elevating the blood sugar. Adrenal hormones of the cortisone group can have the same effect. Sometimes, to save a patient from one of the complications of diabetes such as blindness, it is worth while to destroy part of the pituitary gland (*hypophysectomy*) to reduce the level of growth hormone production.

In a few cases of diabetes, antibodies to insulin have been found, and it has been suggested that in these cases diabetes is an auto-immune disease.

Diabetes, then, may be due to insufficient insulin production, to insulin antagonists such as growth hormone or to anti-insulin antibodies. In some cases yet another mechanism may be responsible. It is possible that in some people a genetic abnormality exists in which the mechanism whereby sugar enters the cells is defective. If this is proved, then some cases of diabetes could be regarded as inborn errors of metabolism affecting all the cells of the body. In such cases, high levels of insulin might be required to stimulate the defective sugar-transporting mechanism into vigorous activity.

There are thus at least four possible ways in which diabetes may be caused, and others may be discovered in the future. In each case the blood sugar level is high, and the cells are starved of sugar due to a defect in the transport of sugar through the cell membrane.

Diabetes is often divided into two types. The Juvenile-onset type occurs in adolescents and is often severe enough to require insulin injections. The other type is called Maturity-onset diabetes and is usually milder. It occurs in middle-aged persons and may be controlled without insulin injections. Both types are partly due to multifactorial inherited gene defects (see page 62).

THE CHEMICAL AND OTHER EFFECTS OF DIABETES

The untreated diabetic has a high level of blood sugar. Often this concentration of sugar exceeds the capacity of the renal tubules to reabsorb it, and *glycosuria* occurs.

Glucose in the urine impairs the reabsorption of water from the renal tubules, and the volume of urine is increased (*polyuria*). This may produce dehydration unless the patient drinks a proportionately large amount of fluid (*polydypsia*).

In diabetes, the tissue cells are deprived of the glucose that they require to produce energy. The only other source of energy that the cells have is from the metabolic breakdown of fat. This utilisation of fat may show as wasting and weight loss. In the absence of glucose, fats cannot be completely metabolised, and they can only be broken down as far as the aceto-acetic acid stage. In diabetes, aceto-acetic acid and similar chemicals called ketones accumulate in the blood and appear in the urine, and they give a curious 'pear drop' smell to the patient's breath.

DIABETIC COMA

Sometimes the first indication of diabetes is a diabetic coma. This occurs due to sugar starvation of the tissue cells, a circumstance to which the brain cells are particularly sensitive as they rely almost entirely on sugar for their energy supply. Patients in diabetic coma are dehydrated, with 'air-hunger' due to acidosis and they may have a detectable 'pear drop' smell to their breath. The urine contains ketones and sugar, and the blood glucose level is high. These features are important in distinguishing diabetic keto-acidotic coma from coma due to excessive insulin.

COMPLICATIONS OF DIABETES

Insulin and diet control are effective in controlling the blood sugar levels in nearly every case of diabetes, and nearly all diabetics can live normal lives. But even though the blood sugar level is well controlled, diabetics are still liable to vascular complications. In fact, 75 per cent of diabetics eventually die from the effects of one or other of the vascular complications.

The arteries of diabetics are very liable to atherosclerosis, with the attendant risks of hypertension, and coronary or cerebral artery thrombosis. The arteries in the legs are particularly liable to atherosclerosis in diabetics, and they may suffer intermittent claudication or even gangrene due to severe ischaemia.

Changes also occur in the arterioles and capillary blood vessels, most marked in the kidneys and the eyes. In the kidneys, renal failure may occur. Sometimes this is entirely due to changes in the capillaries in the glomeruli, but there may also be kidney damage due to pyelonephritis, as the presence of sugar in the urine facilitates bacterial infection. In the eyes, numerous capillary aneurysms may develop, and these may be associated with so many small haemorrhages and thromboses that the retina is destroyed and the patient goes blind.

In summary then, diabetes may have at least four possible causes, insulin deficiency, insulin antagonists, anti-insulin antibodies or a genetic disorder of glucose transport into the cells. Whatever the cause, the principal defect is a high blood glucose while the cells are starved of glucose. There are four main symptoms, weight loss, thirst, polyuria and weakness or even coma. The four major chemical changes are high blood glucose, glycosuria, acidosis and ketosis. And there are four main groups of complications, atherosclerosis and its effects, gangrene of the feet and legs, renal failure and retinal aneurysms and haemorrhages.

Cystic Fibrosis (Fibrocystic Disease of Pancreas, Mucoviscidosis)

Cystic fibrosis is an hereditary disorder. About one child in every thousand is affected. It is an inborn error of metabolism in which the secretions of several groups of glands are affected. The glands involved are the pancreas, the sweat glands and the mucus-secreting glands which line the bronchial tree.

In the pancreas, the digestive secretion is abnormally thick and sticky. It does not flow readily along the pancreatic ducts into the duodenum, but tends to accumulate within the pancreatic glandular tissue and forms the cysts from which the disease takes its name. The pressure of the cysts causes atrophy, followed by fibrosis in the adjacent pancreatic tissue.

In the bronchi, the secretions of the bronchial glands are also thick and sticky, and not like the normal watery mucus that can readily be propelled upwards by the action of the cilia. In the absence of an adequate upward flow of mucus, lung infections are very common.

In the sweat glands, the main abnormality is that the sweat contains an unusually high quantity of chloride. This can readily be tested, and is a valuable aid to the diagnosis of cystic fibrosis.

The first effects of cystic fibrosis may be seen in the newly-born baby as *meconium ileus*, a form of intestinal obstruction due to mucoprotein in the bowel that cannot be digested due to the absence of normal pancreatic secretion. If the child survives, this hazard may be followed by malabsorption, or by repeated respiratory tract infections.

Tumours of the Pancreas

CARCINOMA

The commonest tumour of the pancreas is a carcinoma. It occurs most frequently in the head of the pancreas, and often arises fairly close to the course of the common bile duct, with the result that obstruction to the flow of bile commonly occurs and the patient gradually becomes jaundiced. There may be abdominal pain or discomfort, but it is usually the jaundice that attracts attention, and in some cases surgical removal of the tumour may effect a cure.

Less commonly, a carcinoma may arise in the tail of the pancreas. In this site there is no jaundice, and the tumour may slowly and silently spread into the adjacent tissues, such as the stomach or large intestine, before causing much discomfort. In these cases, the chances of successful surgical treatment are much less.

INSULIN-SECRETING TUMOURS

Insulin-secreting tumours do very occasionally arise in the pancreas. They are usually benign. They attract attention by the attacks of fainting and sometimes of bizarre behaviour which occur due to the effect of the low blood sugar level on the cells of the brain.

14 DISEASES OF THE GENITO-URINARY SYSTEM

Congenital Abnormalities—Polycystic Kidneys

Proliferative Glomerulonephritis

Membranous Glomerulonephritis
Causes of the Nephrotic Syndrome

Urinary Tract Infection and Pyelonephritis

Schistosomiasis (Bilharzia)

Conditions Associated with Pyelonephritis

Hypertensive Kidney

Renal Failure

Tumours of the Urinary Tract
Renal Carcinoma
Wilm's Tumour
Carcinoma of the Bladder

Diseases of the Prostate
Benign Enlargement
Carcinoma of the Prostate

Diseases of the Testis and Epididymis

Each kidney contains a million or so glomeruli, each of which acts as a complex form of filter to adjust the chemical composition of the blood. Each glomerulus consists of a tuft of capillaries coiled into a little ball (Figure 14-1). Water and small molecules such as sodium salts, urea and inorganic acids pass out from the blood, through the walls of the capillaries and into the spaces round the glomeruli. The blood cells and large molecules such as protein stay behind in the blood. They cannot pass through the capillary walls.

The glomeruli in the two kidneys together produce 180 litres of watery filtrate each day, and this passes down the kidney tubules. The tubules reabsorb 178·5 litres of the water, and the sodium salts, but the urea and the inorganic acids are not reabsorbed and they are carried down into the bladder in the remaining 1·5 litres of water.

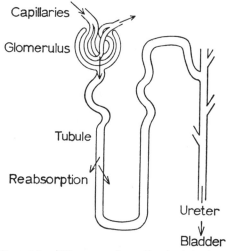

FIG. 14-1 One of the million or so glomeruli and tubules in each kidney

Congenital Abnormalities—Polycystic Kidneys

Polycystic kidneys are the commonest of the various kinds of congenital abnormality that may affect the kidney. In this error of development, it appears that the tubules do not connect up properly with the ureters, and the fluid filtrate that collects in the tubules slowly swells them until they balloon out to form numerous cysts.

The abnormality nearly always affects both kidneys. Any normal tissue in the kidney may be destroyed, either by the presence of the cysts, or by infection, and renal failure eventually occurs.

The various other forms of congenital abnormality likewise lead to renal failure, usually due to infection.

Proliferative Glomerulonephritis

This condition is somewhat similar to rheumatic fever. It occurs in children and young adults, and it follows about three weeks after a streptococcal sore throat. Only a few strains of streptococci are responsible, and some of these strains also produce scarlet fever.

We do not know the precise connection between the streptococci and the glomeruli, but somehow the number of cells in the walls of the capillaries in each glomerulus increases. Each glomerulus swells up and the whole kidney becomes swollen. Often the number of cells increases so much that the blood can no longer pass easily through the glomerular capillaries, and this interference with the blood flow activates the renin-angiotensin system and causes hypertension as described in Chapter 7. There is fever and usually some blood in the urine.

After a few weeks, the patient, in 90 per cent of cases, recovers and the glomeruli completely revert to normal. The hypertension is also transient, as it does not last for long enough for permanent fibrotic contraction of the arterioles to develop.

A few patients die in the acute stage of the disease, and in a few more, the glomeruli do not revert to normal, and they undergo changes that slowly progress until they develop renal failure.

Membranous Glomerulonephritis

The glomerular capillaries are lined by flat cells which lie on a slender membrane, on the other side of which there are epithelial cells which form a network covering the outside of the membrane. The water and other molecules that pass out of the glomerular capillaries to form the filtrate have therefore to pass through or between

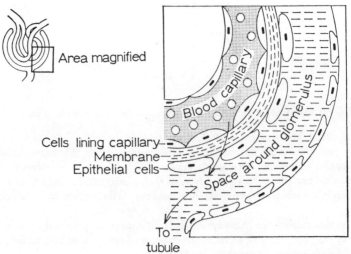

FIG. 14-2 Simplified diagram of part of a glomerulus (magnified many times) to show the position of the membrane between the capillaries and the space around the glomerulus

the capillary lining cells, through the membrane and out through the epithelial cell network into the spaces around the glomeruli (Figure 14-2).

It is this membrane which is affected in membranous glomerulonephritis, and it becomes thickened and very irregular. The changes are so small that they can be seen only by the great magnification of an electron microscope, but the effects are severe. Somehow, protein molecules leak out from the blood and through the damaged membrane into the urine. The change may develop slowly and insidiously and at almost any age. The cause is unknown.

The protein (mostly albumin) can be found in the urine, and the protein leakage reduces the level of the protein in the blood, and, as already described, a low level of protein in the blood is one of the causes of oedema.

The name *nephrotic syndrome* is used when these three features occur together, protein in the urine, low blood protein and oedema. Membranous glomerulonephritis is thus one of the causes of this syndrome.

Eventually the changes lead to renal failure, though steroid treatment may be effective in delaying its onset.

CAUSES OF THE NEPHROTIC SYNDROME
The diseases which may so damage the kidney as to produce protein leakage and the nephrotic syndrome include:
(*a*) Membranous glomerulonephritis.
(*b*) Post-streptococcal glomerulonephritis—in a few cases.
(*c*) Diabetes—in about 10 per cent of all diabetics.
(*d*) Pre-eclamptic toxaemia—which occurs during or just after pregnancy, and in which the nephrotic syndrome is usually reversible.
(*e*) Systemic lupus erythematosus (Chapter 3).
(*f*) Amyloidosis (Chapter 6).

Urinary Tract Infection and Pyelonephritis

Infections of the urinary tract; that is the kidneys, ureters, bladder and urethra, are common. In most parts of the tract, an infection can clear up and leave behind little residual damage, but any infection which reaches the kidney causes permanent damage, with destruction of some of the complex kidney tissue. This is a serious matter, and as the urinary tract is a continuous system of tubing, it is all too frequently possible for infection to spread from one area, such as the bladder, into the kidneys.

Bacteria in the urine cannot effectively move by themselves from place to place, but they may be passively carried by movement of the urine. Normally the flow of urine is downwards, and this tends therefore to remove any bacteria to the outside world.

However, any abnormality of the urinary tract may impair the flow. In children, this may be due to congenital abnormalities of the urinary tract. In women, it may be due to pregnancy, or to dysfunction of the muscles at the neck of the bladder, a condition that is sometimes due to previous pregnancies. In men, a similar impairment of flow may be due to enlargement of the prostate, and in men, women and children, calculi or tumours may impair the flow and produce small spaces where the urine is stagnant. In these circumstances, any bacteria present may multiply without hindrance and many varieties of bacteria can exist and multiply rapidly in warm urine. Any infection may lead to the accumulation of pus or of reactive inflammatory tissue which itself impairs the flow of urine. There is thus a connection between stasis or stagnation, obstruction and infection, such that if any one occurs, the other two are likely to follow, and this can be represented thus:

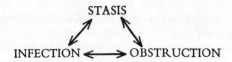

STASIS

INFECTION ⟵⟶ OBSTRUCTION

Bacteria may reach the urinary tract either from the bloodstream or by ascending from the urethral opening. Little is known about how bacteria may enter the bloodstream, but it is certain that the bacteria which normally reside harmlessly in the gut may occasionally be transported through the wall of the gut into the blood and be carried to the kidneys. One of the bacteria that normally reside harmlessly in the gut is called *Escherichia coli*, and this organism is responsible for about 70 per cent of all urinary tract infections.

The perineum is the normal home for a variety of bacteria, particularly in females, and some of these bacteria may be carried up the urethra and into the bladder. It is well known that the passage of a urinary catheter may cause this, and produce cystitis.

In *cystitis*, the lining of the bladder and of the urethra is inflamed, and this causes discomfort, a desire to pass urine frequently and pain as the urine passes down the inflamed urethra. Large numbers of pus cells are present in cystitis, or other infections of the urinary tract, and they may be seen if the urine is examined down the microscope.

In cystitis also, the peristaltic contractions in the walls of the ureters which normally force the urine downwards may be partially reversed, and this reverse flow or reflux may carry bacteria up to the kidneys.

When the kidneys become infected, abscess formation occurs and this is called *acute pyelonephritis*. Such abscesses destroy some kidney tissue, but eventually they heal, leaving small fibrous scars which distort the adjacent kidney tubules. This distortion, by impairing the urine flow, may provide a site for subsequent infections to develop. Repeated infections may destroy a large amount of kidney tissue, and leave a distorted and scarred kidney. This is called *chronic pyelonephritis*, and it is a cause of renal failure and also, due to distorted blood flow, of hypertension.

This lethal disease, chronic pyelonephritis, is still all too common, although it is now largely preventible, by thorough bacteriological investigation and the appropriate antibiotic treatment of every case of suspected infection, and with a strict follow-up of every case to ensure that no bacteria remain after treatment.

Tuberculosis of the kidney is another form of chronic pyelonephritis. It is due to spread of the infection from the lungs via the blood to the kidneys.

Conditions Associated with Pyelonephritis

Hydroureter means widening of the ureter, and hydronephrosis widening of the pelvis of the kidney. These conditions often occur together and are both due to an obstruction further down the urinary tract. In each case the cavity, the ureter or the kidney pelvis, is dilated to form a floppy bag of urine, in which the proper flow of urine cannot take place, and thus infections are common.

Urinary calculi are stones formed of deposits of calcium and other salts. Various factors are involved but it is not known precisely why they form. Stones are usually found in the pelvis of the kidney, where they may seriously obstruct the flow of urine and encourage further infections. They are usually painless, unless all or part of a calculus passes into the ureter, when severe pain occurs, usually accompanied by blood in the urine.

Schistosomiasis (Bilharzia)

One species of Schistosome, the *Schistosoma haematobium*, is endemic in the Nile Valley, but may be encountered in many countries in a huge triangle from Portugal to Bombay to the Cape of Good Hope. *S. haematobium* spends part of its complex life-cycle in a fresh-water snail, and it parasitises man by penetrating the skin from infected water. The parasites migrate until they reach the wall of the bladder, where they cause severe inflammation and haematuria. If the infection is repeated, or persists for twenty years or more as it may, the bladder is eventually contracted by fibrosis, and the associated pain, frequency and haematuria may be very distressing, and subsequent urinary tract infections may cause pyelonephritis and renal failure.

Hypertensive Kidney

Kidney disease as a cause of hypertension has been mentioned previously. But kidney disease can also be a result of hypertension, whatever the cause of hypertension. The arterioles in the kidneys, as elsewhere in hypertension, are contracted, and the blood supply to the glomeruli is reduced. In malignant hypertension, there is also a considerable seepage of fibrin into and through the walls of the kidney arterioles. Many of the glomeruli atrophy as a result of the reduced blood flow, and they are replaced by a clear substance. The whole kidney shrinks and this may further impair the blood flow, and make the hypertension more severe.

Renal Failure

Renal failure is the abnormal biochemical state that exists when the kidneys do not function properly (Figure 14-3). Many of the possible causes have already been mentioned. They include:

(*a*) Congenital abnormalities such as polycystic kidneys.
(*b*) Proliferative glomerulonephritis—in a few cases.
(*c*) Membranous glomerulonephritis and the other causes of the nephrotic syndrome listed previously.
(*d*) Pyelonephritis.
(*e*) Hypertension (especially malignant hypertension).

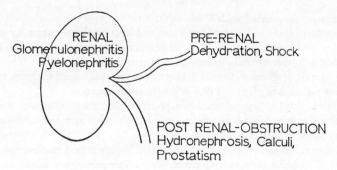

Effects

Blood urea rises
Acidosis - Inorganic acids, H^+ and NH_4^+ retention
Sodium retention
Phosphate retention and calcium loss
Water - Polyuria and polydypsia
Anaemia

FIG. 14-3 Renal failure

The biochemical changes involve:

(a) *Urea*—The blood urea level is raised, and renal failure with a very high blood urea is sometimes called uraemia.

(b) *Water*—A large volume of urine is passed in an attempt to make up for the poor filtration and reabsorption, and the patient requires a large amount of water to drink.

(c) *Acid*—The disposal of inorganic acids is poor and this causes acidosis (page 6).

(d) *Sodium*—The reabsorption of sodium is poor, and sodium salts are lost into the urine.

(e) *Drugs*—Many drugs are commonly excreted through the kidneys, but in renal failure they accumulate in the body and may reach dangerous levels.

These biochemical changes affect all the cells in the body. The effects include anaemia which is nearly always present: deep breathing, as the lungs blow off more carbon dioxide to compensate for the inorganic acid increase; coma or other effects on the brain; and loss of calcium from the bones. Resistance to infection is very poor, and any infection such as bronchopneumonia is usually fatal.

The only salvation for such patients is kidney transplantation or renal dialysis on an artificial kidney machine.

Tumours of the Urinary Tract

RENAL CARCINOMA

A renal carcinoma (sometimes called a hypernephroma) may develop in the kidney tissue. It is less common than a tumour of the bladder, and much less common than tumours of the bronchi, stomach or large intestine. The usual findings are loin pain, a mass in the flank and blood in the urine. This blood in the urine is painless, and painless haematuria always requires thorough investigation as it often indicates a tumour somewhere in the urinary tract. Renal carcinoma tends to spread along the veins and typically it causes rounded 'cannonball' secondary tumour deposits in the lungs.

WILM'S TUMOUR
This unusual tumour of the kidney tissue is one of the few tumours that develop in children, others being retinoblastoma in the eye and neuroblastoma in the brain.

CARCINOMA OF THE BLADDER
Tumours may develop in the epithelium lining the urinary tract, and this occurs most commonly in the bladder, but similar tumours may develop in the pelvis of the kidney or in the ureters. They usually start as papillary growths which may be benign to begin with, though it is possible that they would all become malignant and give rise to metastases if untreated. In the recent past, aniline dye workers were particularly liable to develop these tumours.

Diseases of the Prostate
BENIGN ENLARGEMENT
The prostate is a gland that surrounds the urethra just below the bladder. It makes a watery fluid which is released with the spermatozoa in sexual intercourse. In men over the age of 50, the gland very often enlarges, and sometimes the enlargement obstructs the flow of urine from the bladder and causes infections to develop or hydroureter and hydronephrosis.

CARCINOMA OF THE PROSTATE
Cancer of the prostate is quite common. It develops in men over the age of about 60, and sometimes the patients are much older. The tumour usually develops right at the back of the gland. This sometimes causes obstruction of the urine flow, but often the tumour is first noticed due to secondary tumour deposits, which very often develop in bones and cause pain in the bones. A curious feature of these tumours is that treatment with the female hormone *stilboestrol* is often effective in causing the tumour to become much smaller, but not, unfortunately, to disappear entirely.

Diseases of the Testis and Epididymis
Inflammation of the testis may be due to injury. It may also occur in young men who develop mumps after puberty. Usually the inflammation subsides, but occasionally there is residual fibrosis in the testis, and very occasionally this causes sterility.

Most tumours of the testis are either seminomas or teratomas. A seminoma is a tumour of the tubules that form the spermatozoa. A teratoma is thought to arise from a primitive sex cell. It is a peculiar tumour in that it develops into a variety of structures such as glands, thyroid tissue, alimentary tract epithelium and other tissues. Both these tumours are malignant and they often spread to distant sites in the body.

The epididymis is a common site for infection by the venereal disease Gonorrhoea, and this may sometimes cause scarring and sterility.

Between the testis and the scrotum, there is a double layer called the *tunica vaginalis*. Fluid may collect in the tunica vaginalis and this condition is called hydrocoele. Sometimes it follows infection, and occasionally it is due to a tumour in the testis, but very often there is no apparent cause.

15 *DISEASES OF THE BREAST*

Cancer of the Breast

Other Causes of Lumps in the Breast

Cancer of the Breast

Cancer is by far the most serious of the diseases of the breast, and breast cancer is one of the commonest cancers in women. It occurs in men, but only rarely.

In women, cancer is most commonly seen between the ages of 30 and 60. It is much more likely to occur in the breasts of single women and others who have never had the opportunity to breast-feed any children. In this respect, it is the opposite of the cervix of the uterus, in which cancer is more likely to occur in women with a busy sex life. In the breast, the more work it does the smaller is the chance of breast cancer developing subsequently. As Boyd points out, the cow has the most hard working of all mammary glands, and it never develops cancer.

Early diagnosis is important in breast cancer. Usually the first sign of cancer is a lump in the breast, but it is important to be aware that there may be other early indications of cancer such as asymmetry of the breasts, retraction of the nipple by underlying tumour, bleeding or discharge from the nipple, or the nipple may become roughened, reddened or ulcerated, a condition known as Paget's disease of the nipple.

Cancer may develop in any part of the breast. The tumour slowly enlarges and strands of tumour tissue extend and infiltrate the tissue nearby. The word cancer means crab and this name was used by the ancients because the strands of tissue infiltrating the breast resembled the claws of a crab. The tumour is usually firm and hard, although it develops from soft glandular tissue, and this is because, for some unknown reason, the tumour tissue is usually accompanied by a proliferation of fibrous tissue.

The tumour is malignant. It commonly spreads to the lymph nodes in the axilla. It may also spread by the bloodstream, and this may account for the tumour metastases found in the lungs, liver, bone marrow, brain and elsewhere.

Viruses have been shown to play an important part in causing breast cancer in animals. It is quite possible that they do the same in humans, but the evidence so far is only suggestive. For instance, the serum from women with breast cancer has been shown to suppress the development of breast cancer in animals. This might be due to an antibody in the serum formed by the women against a breast cancer virus.

In animals, breast cancer does not develop if there is a deficiency of oestrogenic hormone in the blood, and this is probably true also of humans. It is sometimes not only the development of breast cancer but also the continued growth rate of the tumour cells which is dependent of oestrogen levels. The growth rate of the tumour cells can sometimes be reduced by removing the sources of oestrogens, the ovaries and the adrenal glands. Unfortunately, the benefit to the patient is usually only transient as after a little while the tumour cells start to multiply again, in the absence of oestrogens.

Other Causes of Lumps in the Breast

Mammary dysplasia is even commoner than cancer as a cause of a lump in the breast. The condition is so common that it can be seen down the microscope to some extent in nearly every breast examined at autopsy, but does not always produce a lump that can be felt.

Although it is so common, we do not know what causes it, though it may perhaps be associated with abrupt changes in the levels of various hormones, such as may occur following abortion, or in the suppression or premature cessation of lactation.

Mammary dysplasia is a combination of cyst formation and fibrous tissue proliferation. Other changes are seen down the microscope, but these are the main ones. The cysts account for the lumps that are felt. They are often multiple and cause areas of lumpiness, often affecting both breasts at once.

Another cause of a lump in the breast is a benign tumour called a *fibroadenoma*, which is most commonly seen in women of a younger age-group than is common with carcinoma, 20 to 40. The tumour is a hard rubbery ball of up to about 5 cm diameter, composed of fibrous tissue enclosing a few glands. It is entirely benign, and the surgeon can usually peel the tumour out from the surrounding breast tissue, rather like removing a stone from a plum.

Sometimes the ducts that convey the milk from the breast glands to the nipple become blocked and swollen (*duct ectasia*), and this also may give rise to a lump in the breast. Sometimes the blockage is due to a small benign *papilloma* in the duct. Occasionally the blockage proves to be a small *intra-duct carcinoma*.

It will be apparent that a lump in the breast may be due to cancer, but more commonly turns out to be due to one of the other causes mentioned. However, all such lumps are treated as if they were cancer until proved otherwise. Early diagnosis is important as two out of three breast cancer patients can be saved if the diagnosis can be made before the tumour starts to spread to the lymph nodes.

16 DISORDERS OF THE ENDOCRINE GLANDS

THE THYROID GLAND
Goitre

Hyperthyroidism (Thyrotoxicosis)

Thyroid Tumours

Hypothyroidism

Cretinism

Myxoedema

THE PITUITARY GLAND

THE ADRENAL GLAND
The Adrenal Cortex

The Adrenal Medulla

THE PARATHYROID GLANDS

The endocrine glands include the pituitary, the thyroid, the parathyroids, the adrenals and parts of the testis, ovary and pancreas. They all secrete hormones into the bloodstream which act as chemical messengers, to modify and to some extent control the chemical activities of the cells of the body. They can all be affected by disease processes, and we have to consider the alterations that may occur in both the form and the function of the endocrine glands as a result of disease. If the form of a gland is abnormal, it is usually a matter of benign enlargement or malignant tumour. If the function of a gland is abnormal, there may be too much hormone production or too little. Sometimes both form and function are affected by the same disease process.

THE THYROID GLAND

The thyroid may be taken as an example to illustrate how the endocrine glands may be affected by disease. A few of the commoner disorders of the other endocrine glands will be mentioned later. (The endocrine functions of the pancreas are dealt with in Chapter 13).

Goitre

A goitre is a change in the form of the thyroid gland, an enlargement which produces a swelling in the neck. The patient may ask for something to be done about it as it looks unsightly, and he cannot fix his collar. Occasionally the enlargement presses on an important structure in the neck, such as one of the veins or one of the nerves that control the vocal cords in the larynx, and then treatment becomes imperative.

The commonest variety of goitre is a simple colloid goitre. It occurs in areas of the world such as the mountains of Switzerland and the Himalayas or in any other area where the soil is poor in iodine. Iodine is one of the principal constituents of the thyroid hormone thyroxine, and the enlargement of the thyroid in simple colloid goitre is a form of compensation, in an attempt to maintain the output of thyroxine in the face of an inadequate supply of raw material. Those who have visited the Salzkammergut region of Austria may have noticed that many of the older people have goitres, especially the women. The younger people do not, and this is because they have taken extra iodine in the form of iodised table salt, a remedy for iodine deficiency that was not introduced until after the older people had already developed their thyroid enlargements.

Hyperthyroidism (Thyrotoxicosis)

Hyperthyroidism is overactivity of the thyroid, with an overproduction of thyroxine. Excess thyroxine stimulates all the cells of the body into abnormally rapid activity. The patient is nervous, anxious and easily upset. The heart beat is rapid. Heat production by all the cells of the body is increased, and the patient may find it too hot indoors. There may be considerable weight loss. Even bowel activity is increased and defaecation may be very frequent.

The excessive function of the thyroid is often accompanied by a moderate goitre, but in hyperthyroidism it is the abnormal function rather than the goitre which is important, on account of the distressing changes it causes. Protrusion of the eyeballs is a curious feature that is often present. The combination of hyperthyroidism, goitre and exophthalmos is called Graves' disease.

Hyperthyroidism is probably due to some stimulator substance circulating in the blood. Overproduction of the thyroid stimulating hormone (TSH) produced by the pituitary gland was at one time suspected, but there is little evidence to incriminate it. Two substances called Long Acting Thyroid Stimulator (LATS) and Human Thyroid Stimulating Immunoglobulin (HTSI) have been found in the blood of some hyperthyroid patients. Little is yet known of how or where they are formed, but it seems very likely that one or both of these substances is responsible for hyperthyroidism, and also the goitre and exophthalmos of Graves' disease.

Thyroid Tumours

Tumours of the thyroid gland are common enough to be responsible for about one in every five hundred deaths. Little is known about the causes of thyroid tumours, but it is known that ionising radiation increases the number of carcinomas that develop, as was seen in the Japanese atomic bomb survivors.

Thyroid tumours occasionally have the capacity to take up iodine from the blood and make thyroxine, and occasionally hyperthyroidism is due to a functioning thyroid tumour, but this is uncommon. In these cases, the uptake of iodine from the blood can be demonstrated by giving the patient a small dose of radioactive iodine and then measuring the radioactivity of various parts of the body. Most of the radioactive iodine usually finds its way to the thyroid in normal people, but if a functioning tumour is present, there is usually a particularly strong focus of radioactivity on one or other side of the thyroid (a 'hot nodule').

However, most thyroid tumours do not show functional activity, and the anatomical derangements due to tumour growth are the main consideration. Tumours of the thyroid are very variable in their rate of growth, but sooner or later they all enlarge, and may give rise to serious trouble by pressing on the trachea, the nerves to the vocal cords or other important structures in the neck. Tumour spread is usually to the lymph nodes in the neck in the first instance, and further spread may be via the lymphatics or the bloodstream, eventually giving rise, if untreated, to tumour deposits in many parts of the body.

Hypothyroidism

Hypothyroidism is a deficiency of thyroxine, the effects of which differ considerably, depending on the age at which the deficiency occurs. Hypothyroidism occurs as cretinism in children and as myxoedema in adults.

Cretinism

Normal thyroid function is necessary for normal growth and development. A cretin is a mental and physical dwarf due to deficient thyroxine production. Cretinism occurs in the Alps and Himalayas and other areas where iodine is lacking in the diet, as the infants cannot manufacture enough thyroxine. These unfortunate individuals are just like tadpoles which fail to develop into frogs if they are kept in iodine-deficient water. A few sporadic cases of cretinism are due to a congenital abnormality of the thyroid gland, in which, although iodine may be plentiful, the gland fails to produce an adequate thyroxine output.

A cretin is small and stupid and slow in every movement, and development is very slow. The condition can be treated by injections of thyroid extract if the diagnosis is made early enough. If treatment is started too late, the critical stages of mental and physical development will have passed, and then the poor child can never hope to catch up.

Myxoedema

Myxoedema, like cretinism, is due to a deficiency of thyroxine, but in this case the deficiency does not develop until the patient is adult, and growth and development are complete.

It is mostly middle-aged women who are affected. All the bodily processes, both mental and physical, are slow. The skin is puffy, the speech and pulse are slow, the patient feels the cold and may sit motionless for hours by the fire. The cholesterol level in the blood is raised in myxoedema, and there is a tendency for atherosclerosis to develop.

The basic change is in the thyroid gland, which is infiltrated by large numbers of lymphocytes, the cells concerned in specific cellular immunity. The glandular tissue of the thyroid is gradually destroyed, and is replaced by fibrous scar tissue. This process is an example of auto-immune disease called Hashimoto's disease of the thyroid gland (Chapter 3). Eventually the destruction of thyroid glandular tissue causes a thyroxine deficiency and myxoedema.

THE PITUITARY GLAND

Diseases of the pituitary gland are uncommon, but tumours do occasionally occur. They are all benign, in that they do not metastasise, but they may nevertheless produce widespread changes. A few pituitary tumours are functioning, and produce excessive growth hormone (hyperpituitarism). If this happens in childhood and is untreated, the child turns into a giant. If the tumour develops after growth is completed, the patient develops acromegaly, with hands and feet like spades, and a large heavy lower jaw.

Most pituitary tumours are non-functioning. The developing tumour presses on the remaining pituitary tissue and destroys it, creating a deficiency of the several hormones that the pituitary normally produces. The clinical features vary, but they include absence of sexual function, obesity, mental lethargy and stunted growth. The growing tumour enlarges in between the optic nerves and it may first be suspected because of progressive blindness due to pressure on these nerves.

The rare condition known as *Diabetes insipidus* may occur if a tumour presses on and destroys the part of the pituitary gland that produces anti-diuretic hormone

(ADH). The lack of ADH forces the patient to pass litres of watery urine, as the reabsorption of water by the renal tubules is much reduced (Chapter 1).

THE ADRENAL GLAND
The Adrenal Cortex
The adrenal gland is really two different organs, one inside the other. The outer part, the cortex, manufactures three groups of hormones, the aldosterone group, which stimulates sodium retention and potassium excretion by the kidneys, the cortisone-like group and the sex hormones.

Excess adrenal function may be due to a functioning tumour of the adrenal cortex or to hyperplasia. The effect depends on which of the three groups of hormones is most affected. An excess of sex hormones produces premature sexual development in boys, masculinisation of girls and women and little change in adult men. An excess of aldosterone production causes sodium retention in the body and potassium loss. The sodium retention may, at least in part, be responsible for the marked hypertension that develops, and the potassium loss may be the cause of the marked muscle weakness that occurs. Excess of the cortisone-like group of hormones produces the curious combination of features known as Cushing's syndrome, which includes the 'lemon-on-matchsticks' figure, due to fat deposition on the trunk and face and muscle wasting in the limbs.

Adrenal cortical insufficiency may occur acutely in young children due to haemorrhage into the adrenal gland. It may also be seen after bilateral adrenalectomy, an operation sometimes performed in breast cancer cases to remove one of the sources of oestrogenic hormone. The most dramatic change in such cases is the rapid drop of blood pressure, perhaps due to sodium loss associated with aldosterone deficiency.

Chronic adrenal insufficiency is called Addison's disease, and is due either to the gradual destruction of the adrenal cortex by disease such as tuberculosis, or to gradual atrophy and fibrosis in a manner somewhat similar to Hashimoto's disease of the thyroid. Such adrenal atrophy is now the commonest cause of Addison's disease, but it is not known whether the disease has an auto-immune basis or not. The features of Addison's disease include low blood pressure, loss of sodium, muscle weakness and often increased patchy pigmentation of the skin.

It will be apparent that the diseases of the adrenal cortex are complicated by the fact that the cortex produces three different groups of hormones, and that with the adrenal cortex it is the effect of these hormones which is important. Anatomical derangements arising from tumours of the adrenal cortex are rare. Occasionally a tumour develops and it can become very large before being noticed as it can displace the organs into other parts of the abdominal cavity, but eventually the anatomical effects of pressure or of metastases may develop.

The Adrenal Medulla
The Medulla normally forms noradrenaline, a hormone which causes the peripheral arterioles to constrict and this raises the blood pressure. The only condition of the medulla which is common enough to warrant mention here is a tumour called a

phaeochromocytoma. This is a functioning tumour of the adrenal medulla. The excessive amount of noradrenaline that it produces causes a severe hypertension that often fluctuates wildly.

THE PARATHYROID GLANDS

The four small parathyroid glands lie, two on each side of the trachea, behind the thyroid gland. They manufacture and secrete parathyroid hormone, which has the effect of stimulating the movement of calcium into the blood, both by increasing the absorption of calcium from the gut and by removing some of the calcium from the bones.

Hyperparathyroidism is due to a tumour in one or other of the four glands. The excess hormone causes the removal of calcium from the bones, which become weak and deformed. The blood level of calcium is high, and calcium may be deposited in abnormal sites such as the kidney, where it may be seen on X-ray. Much calcium is lost into the urine, and stones may form in the kidney.

Similar changes may be seen in secondary hyperparathyroidism. This condition is secondary to renal failure, in which calcium is lost from the diseased kidney. This loss of calcium tends to lower the level of calcium in the blood, and the parathyroid glands respond by secreting more parathyroid hormone in an attempt to maintain the blood calcium level.

Hypoparathyroidism is rare. It is very occasionally seen if the parathyroid glands are unintentionally removed in a thyroidectomy operation. The deficiency of parathyroid hormone causes a very low serum calcium level which may cause tetany.

17 SOME DISEASES OF BONES, JOINTS AND MUSCLES

BONES
Infections of Bone

Osteomalacia and Rickets

Osteoporosis

Hyperparathyroidism

Bone Tumours

JOINTS
Acute Arthritis

Bursitis

Osteoarthrosis (Osteoarthritis)

Rheumatoid Arthritis

Ankylosing Spondylitis

Gout

MUSCLES
Infections of Muscles

Muscular Dystrophy

BONES

Infections of Bone

The term osteomyelitis strictly applies to infection of the bone marrow, but such infections are seldom restricted to the marrow. The adjacent bone is usually involved, and occasionally the infection extends into the neighbouring joint cavity. Infections of bone are frequently the result of damage to the bone, such as may occur in road traffic accidents or war injuries. Sometimes, however, infection develops in bone without any previous injury, and it is probable that in such cases the infecting organisms have been carried to the bone marrow in the bloodstream from an infected lesion elsewhere, such as a boil, which may have healed long before the bone infection becomes apparent.

Bone infections are often associated with fragments of dead bone. Sometimes the dead bone is the result of previous injury, and sometimes the bone cells die as a result of the action of bacterial toxins. In either case, the presence of dead bone fragments makes it difficult for the organisms to be disposed of. Such infections not uncommonly become chronic and form abscesses which may discharge pus from time to time, into the soft tissues and out through the skin.

An important feature of bone infections, or of any other kind of bone damage in children, is that the bone ceases to grow. This may cause a permanent deformity, such as one leg shorter than the other.

Staphylococci are by far the commonest organisms involved in osteomyelitis but other organisms may cause similar infections, and tuberculosis of bones is still seen. Tuberculous infection of bones arises by bloodstream spread of the bacilli from a site of infection in the lungs. The most commonly infected bones are the bodies of the vertebrae, and this is called Pott's disease. The erosion caused by the tuberculosis bacilli may cause collapse of one or more of the vertebrae, causing a hump-back, and sometimes damage to the spinal cord.

Osteomalacia and Rickets

Osteomalacia and rickets are both due to a deficiency of vitamin D. Vitamin D is present in fish-oil, eggs, butter and milk. The human body can manufacture one form of vitamin D if it is exposed to sunlight. A deficiency of vitamin D causes a reduction in the amount of calcium that can be absorbed by the intestines. Normal bones consist of a scanty network of fibres and cells, between which there are large amounts of calcium compounds. Vitamin D deficiency leaves the bones with a normal soft framework of cells and fibres, but the bones are weak as extensive areas are devoid of the hard calcium compounds.

Osteomalacia occurs mainly in women, particularly during pregnancy, as the developing foetus requires about 20 g of calcium from the mother. In osteomalacia, the soft cellular framework of the bones remains intact, but the deficiency of hard calcium compounds leaves the bones soft, and they tend to be distorted by the weight of the body. The leg bones are bowed, the pelvis is flattened and one or more of the vertebrae may collapse. The teeth may also suffer from the deficiency of calcium.

Rickets is the same condition as osteomalacia, but with the important difference that it occurs in children, whose bones are still growing. In such children, the bones are soft and they are usually bowed or deformed as in osteomalacia. In the long bones of the body, such as the ribs and the bones of the arms and legs, lengthwise growth normally occurs by multiplication of the cells near the ends of the bones. In rickets, these cells multiply, but instead of an increase in length, they produce a mushroom-shaped soft lump at each end of the long bones. The children are stunted and bow-legged and they have rickety knobs on the ends of the long bones. These knobs can be felt on the ribs. Severe rickets is now seldom seen in western countries, but lesser degrees of rickets still occur, as was pointed out by Glasgow's Medical Officer of Health in a recent report.

Osteoporosis

In osteoporosis, as in osteomalacia, the bones are fragile and they show poor calcification on X-ray examination, but there the similarity ends. Osteoporosis is a form of bone atrophy, in which the normal loss of bone is not balanced by the normal formation of new bone. Such bone as there is is normally calcified, but the cellular framework is markedly reduced, and there is simply less bone present than normal.

The change appears simple, but we do not know what causes it. Some people divide osteoporosis into idiopathic (which means, cause unknown) and secondary. Osteoporosis is referred to as secondary when it is associated with immobilisation (e.g. in bed-ridden patients or astronauts), with senile or post-menopausal changes, or with various generalised diseases such as Cushing's syndrome, thyrotoxicosis, starvation or malabsorption. Sometimes treatment of these conditions relieves the osteoporosis, but we do not know what causes secondary osteoporosis any more than we know what causes idiopathic osteoporosis.

Osteoporosis is common in elderly women. It may give rise to considerable bone pain, prolapsed intervertebral discs and sometimes to fractures of the fragile bones.

Hyperparathyroidism

Hyperparathyroidism is mentioned here as the bones show some of the main changes in this condition. Excessive production of parathyroid hormone raises the level of calcium in the blood serum, by increasing the amount of calcium absorbed by the intestines, but also by mobilising calcium from the bones. The calcium tends to be removed from the bones in patches, leaving cystic spaces and weak places in the bones, which may fracture (see also page 149).

Bone Tumours

The commonest kinds of tumours in bones are secondary tumour metastases, from primary tumours originating in the bronchi, breast, prostate or other sites. Multiple myelomas are the commonest of the tumours originating within bone, and they really arise in the bone marrow (Chapter 9). The true tumours of bone, such as osteosarcoma, are less common.

Primary or secondary tumours erode the bones and produce local weaknesses. Sometimes the first indication of the presence of a tumour may be a fracture produced with little or no force, a 'pathological fracture'.

JOINTS
Acute Arthritis
Acute inflammation in a joint may be due to physical damage or bacterial infection. Bacterial infection of a joint cavity is not common, but does occasionally occur, due to bloodstream spread of infection from elsewhere. In pre-antibiotic days gonorrhoea was particularly liable to spread to the joints in this way. Joint infections may also occur by direct spread of infection from an adjacent infected bone, or if an infected needle is used to aspirate or inject into a joint cavity.

Acute inflammation is more commonly due to trauma to a joint. In a sprained ankle for instance, the ligaments and joint capsule are damaged and become acutely inflamed.

Bursitis
The bursae around the knee and elbow joints act as small water-filled cushions between the larger tendons and the bones. Inflammation (bursitis) is most commonly due to a direct blow or pressure on the bursa, such as housemaid's knee. There may be bleeding into the bursa and acute inflammation.

Osteoarthrosis (Osteoarthritis)
Osteoarthrosis is the preferable term for this very common ailment, as it is degenerative rather than inflammatory in nature. It is a degeneration of the cartilage which covers the ends of the long bones and which normally forms a smooth glistening joint surface. In the early stages of osteoarthrosis, the cartilage loses its shine, and it becomes dull and pitted and grooved. Later, the cartilage becomes fissured, and eventually it is worn away to expose the rough bone underneath. The joints look as though the cartilage has simply worn out. The wearing out is probably due to some failure of the nutrition of the cartilage cells.

The knees and hip joints are most commonly affected. The disease tends to develop with increasing age. It is considerably commoner in persons who are overweight, who are exposed to persistent trauma, such as the knees of coal-miners, or who have put abnormal stresses on to a particular joint due to a congenital or other bony deformity.

There is usually movement in even the most severely affected joints, but the pain caused by such movement may be crippling.

Rheumatoid Arthritis
Rheumatoid arthritis is a very common progressive inflammatory condition which may involve many of the joints in the body, and may also involve the tendons and muscles. It has nothing to do with rheumatic fever. It usually starts between the ages of 30 and 40, and women are the victims at least three times more commonly than men. The fingers, wrists and ankle joints are the ones most commonly affected, though the shoulders, elbows, hips, knees and vertebral column may all suffer.

The disease often starts with vague symptoms of fatigue, weight loss and stiffness, followed by pain and swelling in the fingers and other joints. At this stage, the synovial lining of the joints proliferates and forms numerous folds, and there is an intense inflammation. The lining becomes packed with lymphocytes and plasma cells, the cells which are principally concerned in the specific immunity mechanism. Some of the folds of the synovial lining of the joint become stuck down on to the joint cartilage, and gradually the smooth shiny cartilage is encroached upon by synovial lining, inflammatory cells and granulation tissue, and the joint surface becomes rough and shaggy. While this is going on, the muscles around the affected joint often show considerable wasting, and small rheumatic nodules may develop under the skin.

The process is very different from osteoarthrosis, which is a degenerative wearing-out of the joint cartilage. Rheumatoid arthritis is an inflammatory condition, in which synovial lining, inflammatory cells and granulation tissue all proliferate.

An auto-immune basis is strongly suspected in rheumatoid arthritis, and there certainly are abnormalities of the specific immunity mechanism. The serum gamma globulins are increased due to the presence of abnormal antibodies in the blood, particularly the so-called rheumatoid factor. The rheumatoid factor is a large anti-body molecule which has the curious property of reacting with and destroying some normal antibody molecules. The rheumatoid factor is present in the blood of most patients with rheumatoid arthritis. Its presence forms the basis of a useful test for rheumatoid arthritis. It is, however, doubtful whether the rheumatoid factor, or any of the other abnormal antibodies present, have anything to do with causing the disease. It could be that rheumatoid arthritis is primarily due to a cellular form of auto-immunity, as is suggested by the constant finding of large numbers of lymphocytes in the synovial lining of the affected joints. There may also be an inherited tendency to Rheumatoid Arthritis. The fact is that the cause of the disease is unknown.

Ankylosing Spondylitis

This is a rare disease of unknown cause which affects males between 15 and 35 years old. In ankylosing spondylitis, the joints between the vertebrae are ossified, especially around the edges of the joints. The whole spine becomes fused into an inflexible rod, which is painful and stiff and may be deformed. Sometimes the disability is so severe that treatment with a radioactive isotope of phosphorus is justified, although it is known that this treatment may occasionally lead to the development of leukaemia. Sometimes other joints, such as the hips or knees, are involved and they show changes very similar to those of rheumatoid arthritis. For this reason, some people think that ankylosing spondylitis should be considered as a variant of rheumatoid arthritis. Cell tests of the kind used to determine compatibility of tissues for transplantation have shown that nearly all patients with ankylosing spondylitis have one particular cell type labelled HL-A W27.

Gout

Gout is a less common affliction than osteoarthrosis or rheumatoid arthritis. It often presents as a sudden intense pain, with swelling and redness of the first joint of the big toe. The first acute attack is usually followed by sporadic attacks over a period of years, and other joints may be involved. The pain is due to deposits of crystals of uric acid in the joints. The affected individuals are known to have a rather higher level of uric acid in the blood than normal people, but it is not known why this should be. Nor is it known why the big toe is so frequently affected.

Gout occasionally develops in patients with myeloid leukaemia undergoing certain kinds of treatment. The breakdown of the nuclei of large numbers of leukaemic cells in this treatment leads to a rise of uric acid level in the blood, and some of these patients develop gout.

MUSCLES
Infections of Muscles
Muscles are not often infected, except in infected injuries, and in these cases the process of healing is much the same as healing elsewhere. There are, however, two infections which particularly involve muscles, namely tetanus and gas gangrene. Both these kinds of bacteria normally reside in the soil. In necrotic muscle tissue, the organisms multiply and produce exotoxins. War wounds and road traffic accidents, in which soil or dirt may be carried into damaged muscle tissue, are liable to be followed by gas gangrene or tetanus.

In gas gangrene, the *Clostridium welchii* or related organisms multiply and produce a plethora of exotoxins which spread into the adjacent muscles. The toxins kill the muscle cells, and the muscle sugar is broken down chemically to form bubbles of carbon dioxide gas.

In tetanus, the exotoxin of *Clostridium tetani* spreads to the brain and spinal cord, probably by seeping up the nerves in the spaces between the nerve fibres. The toxin abolishes the normal mechanism which damps down the activity of the motor nerve cells. Muscle spasms start, and may eventually involve the whole body in violent and exhausting spasms.

The organisms of gas gangrene and tetanus are ubiquitous in the soil. They infect many wounds, but fortunately only about one in five hundred of the many patients infected develop any signs of either of these diseases. This is partly due to the non-specific and specific defence mechanisms, partly due to the careful cleaning of wounds in hospital and the debridement of dead muscle, and partly due to the widespread use of tetanus toxoid prophylactically.

Muscular Dystrophy
The various kinds of muscular dystrophy form an uncommon group of diseases, all of which have an hereditary basis. They are particularly distressing as they slowly develop in apparently normal children. There is an insidious onset, sometimes with swelling of some of the muscles and this is followed by increasing weakness and wasting which spreads slowly from one group of muscles to another. The muscle cells seen down the microscope are pale, swollen and with some loss of the normal cell structures. Various hereditary biochemical abnormalities have been blamed for the changes seen, but it is probable that the biochemical changes are the effect rather than the cause of the disease, and the basic cause is still not known.

INDEX